DYSARTHRIA
SOURCEBOOK
EXERCISES TO PHOTOCOPY

Also available from Speechmark

Working with Dysarthrics

Sandra J Robertson & Fay Thomson (Young)
Speechmark Publishing/Winslow Press, 1986

DYSARTHRIA SOURCEBOOK
EXERCISES TO PHOTOCOPY

SANDRA J ROBERTSON MSc, DipCST, LLCM
BARBARA TANNER BSc, MCST
& FAY YOUNG MA, DipCST, CCC-SLP

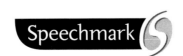

Speechmark Publishing Ltd
Telford Road • Bicester • Oxon OX26 4LQ • UK

*Thanks are due to Val Wilkes for the many
hours she spent patiently typing the manuscript.*

Published by
Speechmark Publishing Ltd, Telford Road, Bicester, Oxon OX26 4LQ,
United Kingdom
www.speechmark.net

© S Robertson, B Tanner & F Young, 1989

First published 1989
Reprinted 1990, 1993, 1994, 1996, 1997, 2000, 2003

All rights reserved. Permission is granted for the user to photocopy and
make duplicating masters for instructional or administrative use only.
No other parts of this book may be reproduced or transmitted in any
form or by any means, electronic or mechanical, including photocopying
and recording, or by any information storage and retrieval system
without written permission from the copyright owners.

002-0355/Printed in the United Kingdom/1030

British Library Cataloguing in Publication Data
Robertson, Sandra
    Dysarthria sourcebook : exercises to photocopy
    1. Articulation disorders – Treatment   2. Speech therapy – Exercises
    I. Title   II. Tanner, Barbara   III. Young, Fay
    616.8'55'06

ISBN 086388 428 8
(Previously published by Winslow Press Ltd under ISBN 0 86388 071 1)

CONTENTS

PREFACE
vii

SECTION 1
ARTICULATION
1

SECTION 2
INTELLIGIBILITY I
37

SECTION 3
INTELLIGIBILITY II
65

SECTION 4
PROSODY I
83

SECTION 5
PROSODY II
113

SECTION 6
PROSODY III
125

ALPHABET CHARTS
130

Sandra Robertson MSc, DipCST, LLCM

Sandra Robertson has been principal lecturer and course director of the BSc Speech Pathology and Therapy course at Manchester Polytechnic since 1983.

After qualifying as a speech therapist from Jordanhill College of Education, Glasgow, she worked for several years in a number of Glasgow hospitals, including the Institute of Neurology and Neurosurgery at Killearn and the Southern General Hospital.

In 1971 she moved to London to take up a lecturing post at the former West End Hospital Speech Therapy Training School, now the National Hospitals College of Speech Sciences. After five years of lecturing, she returned to full-time hospital work as the Chief Speech Therapist for Harrow District Hospitals, based at Northwick Park Hospital. In 1978 she returned to the National Hospitals College of Speech Sciences to lecture and to help develop the BSc in Speech Sciences degree in conjunction with University College, London.

In 1977 she completed an MSc degree in Human Communications, which included research into the long-term effects of anti-epileptic drugs on speech. Her interest in acquired dysarthria has dominated her lecturing, research and clinical activities for a number of years and she has developed and published the *Dysarthria Profile*.

Barbara Tanner BSc, MCST

Barbara Tanner is a speech therapist for the Macclesfield Health Authority. She works with elderly adults on a community basis and with elderly people who are severely mentally ill.

She qualified as a speech therapist from Manchester Polytechnic in 1984 and took up her post at Leighton Hospital, Crewe where she gained experience with a general adult case load and in particular with neurogenic disorders.

In 1986 she became Speech Therapy Clinic Organiser at Manchester Polytechnic which involved supervision and training of speech therapy students and the day to day running of the purpose built on site clinic in the Speech Therapy Department. She moved to her present post in July 1988.

Fay Young (Thomson) MA, DipCST, CCC-SLP

Fay Young qualified from the then West End Hospital Speech Therapy Training School (London) in 1974. Clinical posts in the London area enabled her to gain a wide range of experience with both children and adults in community-based clinics and hospitals.

She developed her expertise in neurogenic disorders at a joint services rehabilitation unit, where the nature of her caseload necessitated consideration of alternative and augmentative communication methods. In 1977 she became involved in the Makaton Vocabulary Development Project, for which she travelled extensively in the UK as part of workshop teams until 1984.

In 1979, she joined the staff at the National Hospitals College of Speech Sciences, where she lectured on acquired speech and language disorders. In August 1984, she left to study at California State University, Hayward, USA and was awarded an MA in *Communication Processes* in December 1985. Her Master's thesis considered the differential diagnosis of the hypokinetic dysarthria of Parkinson's disease, from other dysarthrias.

On returning to England, Fay Young joined the staff of the Central School of Speech and Drama as Year Co-ordinator for the BSc (Hons) Speech and Language Pathology. During her time in this post (February 1986 – December 1988), she was responsible for the organisation and teaching of the curriculum for acquired neurological disorders including clinical practice and examination.

In January 1989, Fay Young took up her current post as District Speech Therapist for Hammersmith & Queen Charlotte's Special Health Authority, based at London's Hammersmith Hospital.

PREFACE

Following the publication of *Working with Dysarthrics* in 1986, the authors received numerous requests for more examples of the exercises contained in that book. *Dysarthria Sourcebook* is a direct response to those requests and should be used in conjunction with the previous publication. The section headings directly relate to some of the parameters assessed and the aims of treatment given for various aspects of dysarthric speech contained in *Working With Dysarthrics*. The areas which usually require a great deal of repetitive practice have been selected and we have tried to provide a wide variety of exercises in each of these areas.

The book is presented in such a way that it can be used directly with the patient. The print is large and clear and each page is arranged in short, manageable groups of exercises or examples. All copyright restrictions have been removed to allow therapists to photocopy any pages they wish patients to take away with them for home practice.

We should stress that this book is not in itself a treatment programme. Rather, we have aimed to provide a workbook that busy practising speech therapists will find useful, labour-saving and therapeutically valuable.

At the end of the book we have included two basic alphabet charts, one in upper case and one in lower case print. From personal experience we have found such a chart (possibly mounted and protected by a clear plastic folder or simply folded to make it easily portable) to be valuable in augmenting a patient's speech. It can either be used to indicate the initial letter of each word, hence increasing intelligibility and slowing rate (Yorkston and Beukelman, *Journal of Speech and Hearing Disorders*, Vol 46, 1981) or in 'impasse' situations it can be used to spell out the whole word.

SR
BT
FY

SECTION 1
ARTICULATION

A	Words with increasingly complex consonant clusters in initial position	3
B	Words with complex consonant clusters in final position	7
C	Words with intervocalic consonant clusters	22
D	Words where consonant clusters change positions and/or complexity	25
E	Words with phonemes in difficult and contrasting combinations	30
F	Short alliterative phrases	33
G	Longer alliterative phrases and rhymes	35

Words with increasingly complex consonant clusters in initial position

A ARTICULATION

eye	lie	fly
ear	leer	clear
and	band	brand
am	ram	pram
and	rand	grand
ink	rink	drink
ill	rill	drill
ice	rice	trice

ace	race	trace
eight	rate	trait
end	send	spend
eye	sigh	spy
oar	four	floor
at	fat	flat
end	bend	blend

ought	bought	brought
it	bit	Brit
eye	pie	ply
eye	pie	pry
are	tar	star
act	tact	tract
air	tear	stare
end	tend	trend

op	top	stop
are	car	scar
eight	gate	grate
oat	goat	gloat

lash	plash	splash
latter	platter	splatter
lay	play	splay

3

ARTICULATION A

rap	trap	strap
ripe	tripe	stripe
roll	troll	stroll
rain	train	strain
ray	tray	stray
rue	true	strew
Ruth	truth	'strewth
ricked	tricked	strict
ride	tried	stride
ring	Tring	string
ripper	tripper	stripper
rate	trait	straight

ram	cram	scram
rag	crag	scrag
rape	crepe	scrape
rue	crew	screw
rum	crumb	scrum
rawl	crawl	scrawl
ream	cream	scream
reed	creed	screed
ripped	crypt	script
rye	cry	scry

sit	spit	sprit
sat	spat	sprat
sane	Spain	sprain
say	spay	spray
said	sped	spread
site	spite	sprite
sigh	spy	spry

A ARTICULATION

sit	spit	split
sign	spine	spline
sing	sting	string
sate	state	straight
sane	stain	strain
sake	steak	strake
sand	stand	strand
say	stay	stray
seem	steam	stream
suck	stuck	struck
soak	stoke	stroke
sole	stole	stroll
sop	stop	strop
sung	stung	strung

seem	scheme	scream
see	ski	scree
seed	skied	screed
sip	skip	scrip
sipped	skipped	script
soup	scoop	scroop
some	scum	scrum
sigh	sky	scry

pay	play	splay
pie	pry	spry
pay	pray	spray
pang	prang	sprang
pig	prig	sprig

cape	crepe	scrape
call	crawl	scrawl
key	Cree	scree
keyed	creed	screed
coo	crew	screw
cooed	crude	screwed
kipped	crypt	script
come	crumb	scrum

ARTICULATION A

Tate	trait	straight
Tain	train	strain
tap	trap	strap
Tay	tray	stray
Tess	tress	stress
two	true	strew
ticked	tricked	strict
tied	tried	stride
tike	trike	strike
tip	trip	strip
tuck	truck	struck
type	tripe	stripe
tipper	tripper	stripper
toll	troll	stroll
tooth	truth	'strewth

Words with complex consonant clusters in final position

B ARTICULATION

mp(s)
mumps
pomp   bump(s)   damp(s)   camp(s)   temp(s)
pump(s)   dump(s)   gamp(s)
vamp(s)   thump(s)   champ(s)   jump(s)   hump(s)
                      chomp(s)   hemp
                      chump(s)

ramp(s)   lump(s)   yomp(s)
lamp(s)   limp(s)

md
aimed   maimed   named
bombed   timed   damned   calmed
          tamed   domed   combed
          teemed   deemed   gummed
                      doomed

farmed   thumbed   shamed   charmed   harmed
foamed   homed
fumed   hummed

warmed   rammed   lamed
wormed   roamed   loomed
          rhymed

nt(s)
ant(s)
meant   pant(s)   taint(s)   can't
mint(s)   pint(s)   tent(s)   count(s)
          paint(s)   tint(s)   gaunt
          bent   dent(s)
                      don't

faint(s) vaunt(s)   sent   shan't   chant(s)
fent(s)   vent(s)   saint(s)   gent(s)

want(s)   rant(s)   lent   haunt(s)
went   rent(s)   lint

ARTICULATION B

nd(z)

and	end(s)			
manned	pond(s)	band(s)	tend(s)	canned
mind(s)	penned	bend(s)	toned	conned
				kind

fanned	vend(s)	thinned	sand	
friend(s)			send(s)	
fend(s)			sinned	
find(s)			sound(s)	
fond			signed	

wand(s)	rand	land(s)
wend(s)	rend(s)	lend(s)
wind(s)	rind	

pt

apt	aped	upped	opt	
mapped	napped			
mopped				
moped				
popped	tapped	dipped	capped	gaped
pipped	topped	doped	cooped	
piped	typed	duped	kept	
	tipped		kipped	
			coped	
sapped	zapped	shopped	chopped	hopped
sopped	zipped	shipped	chipped	hoped
supped		shaped	chapped	hooped
sipped				
wiped	ripped	leapt	yapped	
	rapped	lapped		
	raped	lipped		
	reaped	lopped		

B ARTICULATION

lp/lb
alp
pulp   gulp   yelp   help
bulb

bd
ebbed
mobbed   nabbed
bobbed   dabbed
boobed   tubed   daubed

fobbed   sobbed   jabbed
                  jibbed

robbed   lobbed
ribbed

lt
malt
melt
pelt   belt   tilt   celt   guilt
         built   dealt   kilt
                           cult

fault   vault   salt
felt   silt   hilt
wilt
welt

tl
metal   nettle
petal   battle   tattle   cattle
         bottle   kettle
         Bootle

fettle   settle   chattel
wattle   rattle   little
whittle

ARTICULATION B

ld
old oiled

mailed nailed
mild   kneeled
mulled

paled	bald	tiled	called	geld
piled	bailed	tolled	coiled	guild
palled	boiled	toiled	cooled	gold
		doled		gulled

felled	veiled	sailed	shelled	chilled
fold		soiled		child
foiled		sealed		jailed
fooled				
filled				

wild	railed	lulled	yelled
wailed	riled	lolled	
weald	rolled		
	ruled		

dl
addle

meddle   noodle
middle   needle
muddle   noddle

paddle	beadle	dawdle	coddle
puddle		doodle	cuddle
poodle		diddle	

fuddle   saddle   huddle
fiddle   sidle

waddle   riddle   ladle   yodel

B ARTICULATION

lk(s)
elk(s)	ilk	
milk(s)	balk(s) bulk(s)	talc
silk(s) sulk(s)	hulk(s)	

kl(s)
nickle			
pickle(s)	tickle(s) tackle(s)	cackle(s) cockle(s)	
fickle	shekel(s)	chuckle(s)	hackle(s)

ngk(s)
ink(s)	monk(s) mink(s)			
pink(s) prank(s)	bank(s) bunk(s)	tank(s) plonk(s)	dank	kink(s)
thank(s) think(s)	sank sink(s) sunk	shank(s) chunk(s) chink(s)	jink(s) junk(s)	hank(s) hunk(s)
wink(s)	rank(s) rink(s)	lank link(s)	yank(s)	

gl(s)
eagle(s)				
niggle(s)				
boggle(s) Biggles	toggle(s)	giggle(s) gaggle(s) goggle(s)	jiggle(s) joggle(s) juggle(s)	haggle(s)
wiggle(s) waggle(s)				

ARTICULATION B

mz
aims
maims names
mimes norms
gnomes

poems	booms	times	dams	combs
Pam's	bombs	Thames	dames	coombes
		teems	deems	games
		tomes	dimes	gums
		tombs	domes	

farms	Sam's	shames	charms	harms
fumes	sums		chums	homes
thumbs	seems		James	hums
			Jim's	

worms	rams	limbs
warms	rhymes	lambs
wombs	rooms	looms
	reams	

B ARTICULATION

nz

earns	owns
man's	nines
means	nuns
moons	
moans	

pans	bans	tans	Dan's	cans
pens	buns	tons	dens	cons
pains	barns	teens	dons	guns
puns	bins	tins	dines	
pawns	Ben's	tunes	dunes	

fans	vans	sins	shines	chains
fens	vines	sons	shins	chins
fins	veins			John's
fawns				June's
				Jane's

one's	runs	lens	yearns
wines	runes	lines	
	rains	lanes	
		learns	

ns

ounce	mince	nonce		
pounce	bounce	tense	dense	
			dance	
			dunce	

fence	Vince	since	chance	hence
once	lance			
wince				

ARTICULATION B

nch
inch				
Minch	pinch	bench	tench	conch
munch	paunch	bunch		
	punch			
finch	cinch	haunch		
		hunch		
wench	ranch	launch		
		lunch		
		lynch		

ps
apse	apes	oops		
maps	naps			
mops	nips			
pops	baps	taps	caps	gaps
pips	bops	tops	cops	gapes
pipes		tips	capes	
popes		tapes	copes	
peeps		types	coops	
			keeps	
			cups	
sips	zips	ships	chips	hips
saps	zaps	shops	chops	hops
sops		shapes	chaps	hopes
				hoops
				harps
wipes	raps	laps	yaps	
warps	reps	leaps		
whips	rips	lopes		
	reaps	lips		
	ropes			

sp(s)
asp(s)
| wisp(s) | rasp(s) | lisp(s) | cusp(s) |
| wasp(s) | | | |

ts
| arts | eats | its | oats | eights |

mats	gnats
mits	nets
mates	newts
	knits
	knots
	nuts

pats	bits	tarts	kits	gets
putts	bats	tights	cats	goats
parts	bets	dates	cots	guts
pots	bates	debts	coats	
pits	beats	darts	kites	
puts	buts			
	boots			

fits	sits	shots	chits	hates
fights	seats	shoots	chats	hats
fates	suits	shirts	cheats	huts
vats	sates	sheets	jets	hearts
votes	sets	shuts	juts	heats
vets				hurts

weights	rats	lights	yachts
warts	rates	lutes	
wits	writes	lets	
	roots	lots	
	rots		
	ruts		

ARTICULATION B

st(s)

east	oast			
mast	nest			
mist				
moist				
most				
must				
past	baste(s)	taste(s)	cast(s)	guest(s)
paste(s)	boast(s)	test(s)	cost(s)	ghost(s)
pest(s)	beast(s)	dust(s)	coast(s)	gust(s)
		diced	kissed	
post	bust(s)			
	boost(s)			
	best			
first(s)	vast	chased	jest(s)	haste
fast	thirst(s)		just	host(s)
feast(s)			joist(s)	hoist(s)
fist(s)			gist	hissed
waste(s)	rust(s)	list(s)		
whist	roost(s)	last(s)		
west	rest(s)	lust(s)		
		least		
		lost		
		laced		

B ARTICULATION

ks

aches	arks	auks	ox	
makes	nicks			
mikes	necks			
mucks	knocks			
marks	nooks			
packs	backs	tacks	decks	cakes
pecks	becks	ticks	ducks	cooks
picks	box	takes	dykes	cokes
pikes	books	tocks	docks	kicks
peaks	bikes	tucks	dukes	cox
pox	bakes			
	bucks			
fix	six	shacks	chicks	hacks
fakes	sacks	shocks	checks	hicks
fox	socks	shakes	chocks	hocks
vex	sakes	sheikhs	chucks	hooks
	sex		jacks	
wicks	ricks	licks		
wax	racks	lacks		
works	rocks	locks		
woks	rooks	looks		
	rakes	lakes		
	reeks	leaks		

sk(s)

ask(s)	Esk	mask(s)
musk	task(s)	desk(s)
bask(s)		disc(s)
busk(s)		dusk

Thirsk   husk

whisk(s)	risk(s)
	rusk(s)

ARTICULATION B

bz
ebbs

mobs	nabs			
	knobs			
	nibs			
pubs	bibs	tabs	dabs	cabs
	bobs	tubs	debs	cubs
	boobs	tubes	daubs	cubes
	Babs			
fobs	sibs	jobs		
fibs	sobs	jabs		
	subs	jibes		
ribs	labs			
robes	lobs			
robs	lobes			
rubs				

dz

adds	odds	Ides	odes	aids
mods	nods			
moods	needs			
modes	nudes			
maids	nodes			
pads	bids	tides	dad's	kids
pods	beds	toads	duds	cads
	buds	Ted's	dudes	goads
	bides			gods
	bodes			goods
	bands			guides
	bards			

B ARTICULATION

dz

wads	roads	lads
weds	rids	lids
weeds	rides	loads
wards	reeds	leads
words		
woods		
wades		

zd

eased	oozed	mazed	nosed

dozed	gazed
dazed	

phased	sized	hosed
fizzed	seized	
fused		
raised		

gz

eggs	mugs	nags		
pigs	bags	tags	dogs	cogs
pegs	begs	tugs	digs	kegs
	bugs			gags
	bogs			

figs	sags	chugs	jugs	hugs
fags			jigs	hogs
fogs			jags	hags

ARTICULATION B

lz

ails				
awls	owls	eels	isles	ills
mauls	kneels			
miles	nails			
mills	knolls			
males				
moles				
meals				
mules				
palls	balls	tails	calls	galls
peels	bells	tells	kills	girls
piles	bowls	tills	keels	goals
pills	bulls	tiles	coals	ghouls
pulls	bills	tools	curls	gulls
poles	bales	toils	cools	gills
pales		dolls	coils	gales
		dells	cowls	
		dulls	culls	
fells	vials	sills	shawls	holes
falls	voles	sells	shells	hulls
files	vales	seals	chills	hurls
feels		souls	Jules	hails
foals		soils	Jill's	
fills				heels
furls				hills
fails				halls
fools				
walls	riles	lulls	yawls	
wails	rules		yells	
wools	rills			
wiles	reels			
wills	rails			
wheels				

B ARTICULATION

fs
ifs	oafs			
muffs				
miffs				
puffs	toffs	doffs	coughs	
buffs	tiffs		cuffs	gaffes
chaffs	reefs	laughs		
	ruffs			
	roofs			
	refs			

vz
eaves	ives			
moves	knaves			
	knives			
paves	doves	caves	gives	
	dives	coves		
	Dave's			
fives	saves	shaves	chives	hives
	sieves	shelves	jives	hooves
		shoves		haves
				heaves
				halves
wives	raves	lives		
waves	roves	loves		
		leaves		
		loaves		

ARTICULATION C Words with intervocalic consonant clusters

mp
ampere	umpire	empire	impel
			impale
			impair

pamper	tamper	damper	camper
bumper	temper	dumper	compare
			compass
			campus

vampire	simper	jumper	hamper
thumper	shampoo		

whimper	rampart	limper	yomping
	romper	limpet	
	romping	limping	

mz
crimson	damson	whimsical	flimsy
clumsy			

pt
adapter	interrupted	helicopter
Anaglypta	peremptory	chapter

lp
culpable	palpable	gulper	helper
		gulping	helping

ARTICULATION

st

Easter	austere	aster	assistant
master	nasty		
mister	nesting		
muster			
poster	basting	tasty	castor
pastor	boasting	tester	coaster
pasting	boosting	testing	custard
pastime	Bisto	toaster	gusty
		toasting	
		duster	
		dusting	
		disaster	
faster	vaster	sister	hasty
feasting	vista	zestier	hustings
fester			hosting
foster			hostage
wasting	rusting	lasting	yeasty
wastage	resting	lusting	yesterday
	roasting	listing	
	roosting		

sk

asking	Eskimo	masking	
askance		musky	
basking	tusker	dusky	casket
busking	Tosca	disco	
basket	Tuscan		
biscuit			

ARTICULATION C

sp

Aspel	passport	gospel	Hispaniola
		gasping	
especially			
waspish	rasping	lisping	

s(t)m

postman	dustman	Christmas	gasman
busman			chessmen

Words where consonant clusters change positions and/or complexity

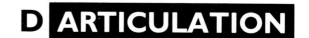

pl

plain	explain	complain	
pleat	deplete		
ply	reply	imply	comply
place	replace	displace	
play	replay	display	
please	displease		
pleasure	displeasure		

pr

prize	apprise	surprise	
print	reprint	imprint	
praise	appraise	reappraise	
present	represent		
press	repress	compress	express
prove	approve	reprove	improve
probate	reprobate		
prudent	imprudent		

bl

blaze	emblazon
blind	purblind
blown	overblown

br

brace	embrace
broil	embroil
broad	abroad
bridge	Cambridge
bred	inbred

ARTICULATION D

tr

trace	retrace	
tract	retract	contract
train	retrain	entrain
transitive	intransitive	
trap	entrap	
treat	retreat	entreat
tray	ashtray	
trench	retrench	entrench
trite	contrite	
trait	nitrate	concentrate

dr

dress	address	redress
drake	mandrake	
drill	mandrill	
drum	eardrum	
drop	teardrop	

kr

craft	aircraft	handicraft

kl

close	enclose	disclosure
clip	unclip	
claim	disclaim	disclaimer

gr

grade	regrade	upgrade	retrograde
gram	milligram	phonogram	telegram
grate	ingrate	ingratiate	
grieve	aggrieve		
grave	engrave		
grin	chagrin	peregrine	
group	regroup	subgroup	

gl
glass	wine glass
glue	igloo

sp
spur	hotspur		
span	outspan		
spare	despair		
special	especial		
spectacled	bespectacled		
spell	gospel		
Spence	dispense	suspense	
spy	espy		
spire	aspire	respire	inspire
spite	despite	respite	in spite
spoil	despoil		
spoke	bespoke		
spouse	espouse		

spl
splay	display
splendour	resplendent

spr
spray	respray	osprey
spread	bedspread	
spring	bed spring	

ARTICULATION D

st

stable	unstable	constable
stack	haystack	
staff	distaff	
stage	upstage	on stage
stall	bookstall	
stand	bandstand	
start	restart	upstart
stay	mainstay	outstay
steady	unsteady	
stain	abstain	
step	doorstep	
steer	austere	
steroid	asteroid	
stick	joystick	slapstick
still	instil	
sting	bee sting	
stir	bestir	
stitch	unstitch	
stock	restock	
stocking	bluestocking	
store	restore	
stuck	unstuck	
stump	tree stump	

str

straddle	bestraddle	
strain	restrain	constraint
strap	unstrap	
stream	upstream	downstream
strew	construe	
strict	restrict	constrict
strike	on strike	
struck	star struck	construction
strudel	apple strudel	
strung	restrung	
stretch	outstretch	

sk
scale	descale	
scant	descant	
scape	escape	landscape
scarp	escarpment	
scope	telescope	gyroscope
score	earth's core	
Scot	Ascot	
skit	biscuit	
scar	mascara	
scuttle	coal scuttle	
scutch	escutcheon	
skate	ice skate	roller skate

sky
skew   askew

skr
scream	ice cream
screen	smoke screen

sn
snack   bar snack

sl
slam	grand slam
slaw	coleslaw
sleep	asleep
sling	gin sling
slide	backslide

ARTICULATION E

Words with phonemes in difficult and contrasting combinations

lime	loam	mill	mile
loam	loom	mole	meal
line	Len	nil	Nile
lean	loan	knoll	kneel
lit	let	till	tall
light	loot	tile	tool
lot	late	tall	tale
lip	lop	pal	pool
lap	leap	pall	pail
loop	leap	pile	pill
lab	lob	ball	bell
lid	lad	deal	dell
lied	load	dole	dill
laid	lord	dull	dale
lick	lack	kill	call
lack	lake	kale	coal
look	leak	cool	keel
like	lack	Kyle	curl
lag	leg	gall	girl
lug	log	goal	ghoul
leg	league	guile	gull
laugh	leaf	feel	foal
life	loaf	foul	fell
love	lave	vole	vile
lave	live	veal	vale

ARTICULATION

lass	loose	sail	sell
loss	lice	seal	sale
lush	lash	shall	shell
lash	leash	she'll	shoal

latch	lych	chill	churl
ledge	lodge	gel	jewel

some	same	miss	mess
Sam	seem	mass	mice
son	sin	ness	nice

sip	soap	pass	puss
sib	sob	bus	boss
sit	sat	toss	Tess
soot	set	terse	toss
sick	sack	kiss	curse
suck	seek	case	Cass
sag	sog	gas	goose

shame	sham	mush	mash
shin	shine	nosh	gnash
ship	shape	posh	push
shot	shoot	tosh	'tache
shack	shock	cash	cosh
she'll	shell	leash	lash

chip	chap	pitch	patch
chop	cheap	peach	pouch
chick	chalk	ketch	catch
chit	chat	touch	teach
chum	Cheam	much	match
chine	chin	notch	natch
chaff	chafe	fetch	fitch

ARTICULATION E

farm	form	miff	muff
fib	fob	buff	beef
fat	feet	toff	tough
fag	fog	gaff	goof
fall	fell	leaf	laugh
jam	gem	Madge	midge
jap	jeep	podge	pudge
Jill	gel	lodge	ledge

Short alliterative phrases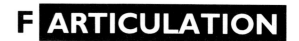

Mince meat on Mondays
Ninety-nine names
Wee Willie Winkie

Play the piano
Peace and pardon
Pick up a penguin
Peaches pears and pineapples
Pretty Polly Perkin

Birds and bees
Buy Bob's bread
Black Beauty
Buy a bun
Billy Bunter
Big bad boy

Tiny Tim
Two pounds ten pence
Tom tied the tie
Donkey Derby
Dundee's dry dock
Dig down deep

Country cottage
Cream crackers
Kick the cat
Cup of coffee
Court of kings and queens

King's Cross
Cross-eyed Clare
Crazy crosswords
Crunchy corn flakes
Good gifted girl

ARTICULATION F

Frozen food
A foggy frosty Friday
Fair fat and fifty
Foreign fields of France
Fly the flag of freedom
Fellow feeling

Sit on a seat
Stop and stare
City slicker
Sly salesmen
Susan's see-saw
Sand sea and sun

Sing something simple
Sprint swiftly
Scrimp and scrape
Spring is sprung
String is strong
Elastic is strong and stretchy

Ship to shore
All ship-shape
A shrimp is a shell fish
Shrieking shrew
A shetland shawl

Chop and change
Church bells chime
Cheerful Charlie
Jumping Jack

Robin redbreast
Hitch-hike to Holland
Unique New York

Longer alliterative phrases and rhymes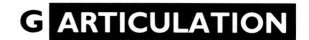

Any noise annoys an oyster

Wake up on a wet windy wintry Wednesday

Wishy-washy Wilfred wished to win a washing machine

A packet of popcorn, please

Oporto's a port in Portugal

A proper cup of coffee from a proper copper coffee pot

How many cookies could a good cook cook?

Three Scottish thistles in the thicket

Forty-four famous fishermen fried flat fish

Five frantic frogs fleeing from the pond

He sold some snowdrops on Sunday

Seventy shivering sailors stood silently

Sheila and Sharon washed the dishes

Shadows shade the sheltered shore

Harry's hedgehog's hiding in the high hedge

ARTICULATION G

'Good, better, best,
 Never be at rest,
 Till your good is better,
 And you better best.

Whether the weather be fine
Or whether the weather be not.
Whether the weather be cold
Or whether the weather be hot.
We'll weather the weather
Whatever the weather,
Whether we like it or not.

To sit in solemn silence
In a dim dark dock
Awaiting the sensation
Of a short sharp shock
From a cheap and chippy chopper
On a big black block.'

(WS GILBERT)

'In short, in matters vegetable, animal and mineral
I am the very model of a modern Major-General.'

(WS GILBERT)

SECTION 2
INTELLIGIBILITY I

The exercises which follow in this section have been designed to assist in the building up or extension of intelligibility.

A	**Words with increasing number of syllables, using the same root**	39

B	**Words with increasing number of syllables**	47

*Words with **two** syllables/47*
*Words with **three** syllables/51*
*Words with **four** syllables/54*
*Words with **five** syllables/56*
*Words with **six** syllables/58*

C	**Phrases and sentences with increasing number of syllables**	59

*Phrases/sentences with **three** syllables/59*
*Phrases/sentences with **four** syllables/60*
*Phrases/sentences with **five** syllables/61*
*Phrases/sentences with **six** syllables/62*
*Phrases/sentences with **seven** syllables/62*
Longer than seven-syllable phrases/sentences/63

Words with increasing number of syllables, using the same root

A INTELLIGIBILITY I

A
aft	after	afternoon
account	accountant	accountancy
accuse	accusing	accusingly
alter	alternate	alternator
awake	awaken	awakening
author	authorise	authorisation

B
boast	boastful	boastfully
ban	banner	bannerman
bound	bounder	boundary
but	butter	buttercup
bat	batter	battering
bit	bitter	bitterly

C
car	carpet	carpenter
count	counter	counterfeit
cab	cabin	cabinet
cam	camber	Camberwell
camp	campaign	campaigner
can	canal	Canaletto
can	candid	candidate
can	candy	candyfloss
cape	caper	capering
cap	captain	captivate
car	carbon	carbonate
care	careful	carefully
corn	corner	cornering
cat	cattle	catacomb

INTELLIGIBILITY I A

Chris	Christmas	Christmastide
clam	clamour	clamouring
cough	coffee	coffeepot
come	comfort	comforting
con	contempt	contemplate
cook	cooker	cookery
cope	coping	copious
count	counter	counteract
cream	creamer	creamery
crust	crusty	crustacean
cute	cutie	cuticle
cure	curate	curator
curse	cursor	cursory
can	cancel	cancellation
cat	catarrh	catastrophe
con	conserve	conservative
calor	calorie	calorific
certain	certify	certificate
circle	circulate	circulation
civil	civilise	civilisation
commerce	commercial	commercialise
construct	constructive	constructively
create	creative	creativity

D

dive	diver	diversion
dine	dining	dining-room
deaf	deafen	deafening
dare	daring	daringly
dog	dogged	doggedly
disc	discuss	discussion
die	digest	digestive
dire	direct	direction
dirt	dirty	dirtiest
disc	disco	discotheque
drag	dragon	dragonfly
dress	dressing	dressing-gown
dip	diploma	diplomatic

A INTELLIGIBILITY 1

dispense	dispenser	dispensable
danger	dangerous	dangerously
deceit	deceitful	deceitfulness
devote	devotion	devotional

E
edit	editor	editorial
elect	elector	electoral
embark	embarking	embarkation
engage	engaging	engagingly
equal	equalise	equalisation
except	exception	exceptional

F
fab	fabric	fabrication
false	falsehood	falsify
fan	fancy	fanciful
fast	fasten	fastening
far	father	fatherhood
feat	feature	featureless
fill	filler	filament
fine	finer	finery
fin	finish	finishing
firm	firmer	firmament
fish	fisher	fisherman
fix	fixate	fixation

fore	forecast	forecaster
for	forget	forgetful
form	formal	formally
found	founder	foundation
freak	frequent	frequency

fright	frightful	frightfully
frost	frosty	frostiness
fun	funny	funniest
faith	faithful	faithfully
fate	fatal	fatalist
finance	financial	financially

INTELLIGIBILITY 1 A

G
gain	gainful	gainfully
guard	garden	gardening
glim	glimmer	glimmering
gloss	glossy	glossier
gold	golden	Goldilocks
green	greener	greenery
grow	grocer	grocery
grace	gracious	graciousness
glamour	glamorous	glamorously

H
herb	herbal	herbalist
hope	hopeful	hopefully
hard	harder	hardier
hand	handy	handier

I
impose	imposing	imposition
inflate	inflation	inflatable
idol	idolise	idolisation
image	imagine	imagination
immune	immunise	immunisation
intent	intention	intentionally
illumine	illuminate	illumination

J
joy	joyful	joyfully
joke	joking	jokingly
juice	juicy	juiciness

K
kid	kidnap	kidnapper
kind	kindly	kindliness
king	kingly	kingliness
kit	kitchen	kitchenette

A INTELLIGIBILITY I

L
length	lengthen	lengthening
long	longing	longingly
live	lively	livelier
laugh	laughing	laughingly
limb	limber	limbering
love	lovely	loveliness
labour	laborious	laboriously

M
man	manful	manfully
mean	meaning	meaningful
might	mighty	mightier
mar	martial	martialling
mourn	mournful	mournfully
mount	mountain	mountainous
moon	moonlight	moonlighting
mark	market	marketing
mat	matter	material
manage	manager	manageress
million	millionaire	millionairess
moment	momentous	momentously
motive	motivate	motivation
mystery	mysterious	mysteriously
melody	melodious	melodiously
monotone	monotonous	monotonously

N
nine	ninety	ninety-nine
new	newsy	newsworthy
night	nightly	nightingale
nation	national	nationalise
neglect	neglectful	neglectfully

INTELLIGIBILITY I A

O

object	objective	objectively
oppose	opposite	opposition
observe	observation	observational
occasion	occasional	occasionally
origin	original	originally

P

pay	paper	papering
pen	penny	penniless
pop	poppy	poppadum
port	porter	portering
part	partner	partnership
pat	pattern	pattering
pain	painful	painfully
play	playful	playfully
peace	peaceful	peacefully
prayer	prayerful	prayerfully
passion	passionate	passionately
pity	pitiful	pitifully
plenty	plentiful	plentifully

Q

quick	quicken	quickening
quiz	quizzical	quizzically
question	questioning	questioningly

R

ration	rational	rationally
real	really	realistic
region	regional	regionally
relate	relation	relationship
respect	respectful	respectfully
regiment	regimental	regimentation

A INTELLIGIBILITY I

S

sale	salesman	salesmanship
sand	sandal	sandalwood
save	savour	savoury
scene	scenic	scenery
sea	season	seasoning
salt	salty	saltiness
seem	seeming	seemingly
sell	seller	sellotape
set	settle	settlement
sing	single	singular
scorn	scornful	scornfully
sleep	sleepless	sleeplessness
strength	strengthen	strengthening
style	stylist	stylistic
sat	satire	satirical
sect	sector	sectarian
sense	sensation	sensational
select	selective	selectivity
science	scientist	scientific
sorrow	sorrowful	sorrowfully
station	stationer	stationery
standard	standardise	standardisation
simple	simplify	simplification
satisfy	satisfaction	satisfactory

T

tot	totter	tottering
tell	telling	tellingly
taste	tasteful	tastefully
thank	thankful	thankfully
thick	thicken	thickening
thought	thoughtless	thoughtlessness
threat	threaten	threatening
truth	truthful	truthfulness
therm	thermal	thermometer
temper	temperament	temperamental
tranquil	tranquillise	tranquilliser
tradition	traditional	traditionally

INTELLIGIBILITY I A

U
use	useful	usefully
unit	unity	unitisation
universe	universal	universally

V
van	vanish	vanishing
verse	version	versatile
vary	variant	variation
very	verity	veritable
visit	visitor	visitation
victim	victimise	victimisation
vocal	vocalise	vocalisation

W
wake	waken	wakening
weight	weightless	weightlessness
wit	witty	witticism
wood	wooden	woodenness
word	wordy	wordiness
work	workman	workmanlike
world	worldly	worldliness

Y
yell	yellow	yellowish
yield	yielding	yieldingly
youth	youthful	youthfully

Z
zig	zig-zag	zig-zagging
zip	zipper	zip-fastener
zoo	zoology	zoological

Words with increasing number of syllables

B INTELLIGIBILITY I

■ **Words with *two* syllables**
▶ *Equal stress*

backlog	booklist	blue-print
dead-heat	dry-lock	first-rate
first-hand	half-price	half-size
half-way	hitch-hike	ice-cream
ill-will	indoors	kick-off
left-off	lifesize	May-queen
meat-pie	mid-on	mince-pie
mint-sauce	misdeed	misspell
misuse	mix-up	non-stop
north-west	oatcake	off-hand
one-eyed	outside	outspread
pea-soup	post-war	pot-luck
prejudge	preview	pre-war
re-arm	re-birth	red-hot
re-dial	relay	remould
reprint	rig-out	roll-top
scot-free	screw-cap	seashore
seesaw	self-will	shipyard
skin-deep	sky-high	snow-plough
snow-white	south-east	south-west
sponge-cake	stone-cold	tail-end
tax-free	third-rate	tiptoe
tiptop	top-coat	trapdoor
two-edged	unborn	unbound
unclean	uncork	uncut
unfed	unjust	unknown
unlike	unpaid	unsigned
untrue	unwell	waist-deep
waist-high	week-end	well-bred
well-known	well-off	wheelchair

INTELLIGIBILITY I B

- **Words with *two* syllables**
- ▶ *Stress on **first** syllable*

abbey	acid	after
airmail	barber	cabin
cabbage	carpet	cheesecake
Christmas	comfort	dagger
doctor	daughter	devil
earning	earthquake	eastern
endless	fabric	fillet
fireman	football	gallant
gammon	habit	haddock
hardboard	headache	highlight
iceberg	igloo	illness
income	infant	inland
insect	jacket	jealous
jolly	journey	keepsake
kestrel	keyboard	kidnap
kipper	label	lacquer
lakeside	lamppost	lampshade
landmark	landscape	language
laundry	leaflet	lifelike
likewise	lipstick	living
magnate	major	matchless
meadow	metal	midnight
mincemeat	moral	mouthful
nanny	nature	necklace
neutral	newborn	nightfall
normal	oatmeal	oblong
oboe	octave	oddment
olive	option	order
ostrich	outlet	outreach
oyster	package	painful
palace	partner	peanut
pewter	phantom	pigeon
pigtail	pillow	pilot
planet	pressure	promise
pupil	purpose	quadrant
quaker	quarrel	quarter
quicken	quiet	rabbit
race-horse	ragtime	railway

B INTELLIGIBILITY I

ransom	rasher	regal
rigid	ripen	river
roadside	rubber	ruby
rugger	runway	sabbath
safeguard	salesman	salmon
sandwich	satin	saucepan
saving	scarecrow	schoolboy
seaweed	sentence	sheepskin
shorthand	silence	slipper
slumber	smokeless	smuggler
snooker	snowdrop	something
soundtrack	spanner	sparrow
speechless	splendid	springtime
suburb	sunrise	sunset
sunshine	tablet	tactful
take-off	tandem	taxi
teacher	tea-leaf	teapot
tea-time	tenant	textile
tooth paste	trumpet	turkey
ugly	upkeep	upper
upright	upward	useless
vaccine	vacuum	valid
valley	versus	very
vicar	villa	voiceless
wagon	waistband	walnut
wardrobe	warehouse	washing
water	welfare	widow
wigwam	windscreen	yellow
yoghurt	youngster	zealot
zebra	zero	zigzag

INTELLIGIBILITY I B

- **Words with *two* syllables**
- ▶ *Stress on **second** syllable*

abduct	abroad	accept
across	again	attack
belong	cadet	degree
defy	discuss	endure
enlarge	enrol	erect
exchange	forbid	foretell
galore	hurray	ignite
impress	impart	impede
include	indeed	inert
infect	lacrosse	lagoon
lament	lapel	machine
maltreat	mankind	migrate
morale	naive	obese
obey	obscure	obsess
obstruct	obtain	offence
opaque	outbid	papoose
parade	parole	partake
perhaps	phonate	pipette
police	pollute	postpone
presume	prevail	prevent
propose	quinine	quintet
racoon	ravine	recite
recline	recruit	regard
regret	relapse	remain
robust	rosette	saloon
salute	sedate	select
stampede	sublime	submerge
subside	sustain	tattoo
technique	themselves	today
to-do	tonight	towards
translate	uncouth	unless
velour	veneer	vibrate
whereas	yourself	

B INTELLIGIBILITY I

■ Words with *three* syllables
▶ *Primary stress on **first** syllable*

accident	atmosphere	bachelor
balcony	breathlessness	bungalow
butterfly	caliper	camera
cabinet	candidate	Capricorn
caravan	criminal	daffodil
deputy	document	dressing-gown
dynasty	easterly	elephant
factory	faculty	fanciful
fearlessly	garrison	glorious
government	gratitude	habitat
handicraft	heavenly	hemisphere
icicle	imitate	increment
indicate	invalid	irony
ivory	jaguar	jelly-fish
jeweller	juvenile	kindliness
kingfisher	kilogramme	lateral
latitude	liberal	limerick
magistrate	magnitude	maintenance
marvellous	matronly	melody
memory	modify	mutiny
natural	neighbourhood	newspaper
northerner	noteworthy	obligate
obvious	octopus	orifice
opening	organist	orphanage
outpatient	overdraft	oxygen
pace-maker	pacifist	pancreas
pantomine	paper-clip	parachute
paragraph	passenger	pedigree
penalty	policy	poverty
presently	publican	punctual
quadruped	qualify	radio
randomise	raspberry	razor-blade
regular	residence	roundabout
saccharine	safety-pin	satellite
scaffolding	scenery	scrutiny
seasonal	shareholder	shopkeeper
shrubbery	signature	silverside
solitude	stamp-duty	stethoscope

INTELLIGIBILITY I B

stockbroker	strawberry	sympathy
tabulate	tailormade	talkative
teenager	telegram	telephone
testament	therapist	thunder-storm
ulcerate	underground	underlay
vacancy	vascular	versatile
vinegar	walking-stick	wall-paper
warranty	weather-proof	wedding-ring
yesterday	zip-fastener	zodiac

▶ *Primary stress on **second** syllable*

abandon	abolish	adventure
banana	collection	department
digestive	diploma	discover
discussion	domestic	efficient
elicit	employer	engagement
expensive	flamingo	gorilla
humanely	hypnosis	ignition
impassive	impression	inhabit
injection	magician	mascara
mechanic	midwinter	mimosa
misguided	narcotic	nocturnal
nostalgic	occasion	opinion
optician	oration	otitis
palatial	parental	percussion
perfection	physician	plum-pudding
pneumatic	prescription	probation
provision	quadratic	quick-tempered
quick-witted	reactor	red-handed
red-letter	redundant	refreshing
religion	remember	retirement
romantic	safari	sarcastic
securely	selection	self-centred
spaghetti	spectator	starvation
stiletto	straightforward	tarpaulin
thereafter	thoracic	tomorrow
torpedo	umbrella	unconscious
unhealthy	unsporting	whenever

B INTELLIGIBILITY I

▶ *Primary stress on **third** syllable*

flannelette	immature	introduce
jamboree	kangaroo	mountaineer
pioneer	re-address	recommend
referee	refugee	tambourine
tangerine	violin	volunteer

▶ ***Three**-syllable words with **two** primary stressed syllables*

overdue	overwork	overwrought
ready-made	re-elect	second-class
self-employed	seventeen	unashamed
underdone	well-to-do	

INTELLIGIBILITY I B

■ **Words with *four* syllables**
▶ *Primary stress on **first** syllable*

busybody	dangerously	favourably
generally	helicopter	kindergarten
laminated	legislative	luminously
methylated	necessary	ominously
onerously	pleasurably	pomegranate
procurator	quarter-master	questionable
radiator	secretary	semi-final
subdivision	supermarket	tantalising
tax-collector	telegraph-pole	television
testimony	tabulated	undercarriage

▶ *Primary stress on **second** syllable*

abbreviate	ability	accompany
ambassador	biologist	bureaucracy
chrysanthemum	directory	discriminate
embarrassing	emergency	euphonium
geography	geranium	grammatical
harmonious	hostility	humidity
illiterate	immunity	impersonate
incompetence	kaleidoscope	locality
magnanimous	majority	medicinal
meticulous	minority	modality
neurologist	normality	numerical
nutritiousness	olfactory	oblivious
obscurity	officially	omnipotent
parameter	particular	pathologist
pedestrian	persistently	philosophy
photographer	plasticity	prosperity
psychology	rapidity	receptionist
ridiculous	satirical	severity
significant	simplicity	sincerity
society	solicitor	spectacular
speedometer	stability	tarantula
theatrical	thermometer	tobacconist
transparency	undisciplined	variety
vivacity	zoology	

B INTELLIGIBILITY I

▶ *Primary stress on **third** syllable*

academic	allocation	circumstantial
comprehension	correspondence	dehydration
disappointment	distribution	expedition
fascination	fermentation	fluctuation
geometric	haemoglobin	hibernation
illustration	imperfection	incarnation
incubation	inexpensive	institution
jubilation	journalistic	laceration
liberation	liquidation	malformation
meditation	meningitis	navigation
nomination	obbligato	operatic
ordination	ostentatious	palpitation
panorama	penetration	penicillin
pentecostal	perforation	periodic
pessimistic	philanthropic	politician
population	preposition	reconstruction
referendum	reproduction	retrospective
segregation	sentimental	superstition
sympathetic	telegraphic	telescopic
termination	therapeutic	transatlantic
ultimatum	ultrasonic	ventilation

▶ ***Four**-syllable words with **two** primary stressed syllables*

• *First and second*

post-graduate   re-educate

• *First and third*

misconception	nonconformist	open-minded
over-anxious	polytechnic	preconception
rediscover	unabated	unbelieving
undecided	understatement	unemployment
unexpected	well-connected	

• *First and fourth*

over-subscribe

INTELLIGIBILITY I B

■ **Words with *five* syllables**
▶ *Primary stress on **first** syllable*

lightning-conductor

▶ *Primary stress on **second** syllable*

commemorative	deliberately	luxuriousness
perambulator	precautionary	professionally
proportionally	unnecessary	

▶ *Primary stress on **third** syllable*

alphabetical	anniversary	cardiologist
disability	disagreeable	documentary
electricity	fundamentally	gynaecologist
hospitality	inappropriate	inarticulate
inconspicuous	inhumanity	international
joviality	legibility	manufacturer
masculinity	methodology	metropolitan
ministerial	nationality	notoriety
occupational	optimistically	ornithologist
orthographical	pandemonium	parallelogram
perpendicular	pharmacologist	polysynthesis
professorial	quadrilateral	revolutionist
similarity	speciality	subjectivity
suitability	supernatural	technicality
theoretical	trigonometry	university

B INTELLIGIBILITY I

▶ *Primary stress on **fourth** syllable*

abbreviation	accommodation	amplification
clarification	classification	communication
denomination	evacuation	exaggeration
extermination	extravaganza	fertilisation
fortification	fossilisation	hallucination
idealistic	justification	legalisation
matriculation	multiplication	notification
organisation	orientation	ornamentation
participation	perpetuation	pronunciation
qualification	ratification	realisation
sanctification	sophistication	specification
subordination	terrorisation	vaporisation

▶ ***Five**-syllable words with **two** primary stressed syllables*

● First and second

  unappetising   uncompromising

● First and third

  hypersensitive   overconfident   radiography
  unaccompanied   unconventional   unidentified

● First and fourth

  holiday-maker   misapplication   non-intervention
  overproduction   predisposition   radioactive
  self-preservation transcontinental

INTELLIGIBILITY I B

■ **Words with *six* syllables**
▶ *Primary stress on **third** syllable*

simultaneously

▶ *Primary stress on **fourth** syllable*

autobiography	co-educational	encyclopaedia
humanitarian	idiosyncrasy	impetuosity
impossibility	inferiority	juxtapositional
ostensibility	paraphernalia	parliamentarian
perceptibility	potentiality	profitability
psychoanalysis	respectability	totalitarian

▶ *Primary stress on **fifth** syllable*

decontamination	disqualification	electrification
identification	militarisation	nationalisation
personification	reconciliation	superannuation

▶ ***Six**-syllable words with **two** primary stressed syllables*

● First and third
  uncommunicative   unprofessionally

● First and fourth
  heterogeneous   radiotherapy   unsatisfactory

● First and fifth
  maladministration   misrepresentation   over-estimation
  rehabilitation   reorganisation   secularisation
  transubstantiation

Phrases and sentences with increasing number of syllables

C INTELLIGIBILITY I

■ **Phrases/sentences with *three* syllables**

Where's the soap?	How are you?
Is this yours?	Black or white?
Where is it?	Here you are.
By the bed.	On the shelf.
By the fire.	On the wall.
In the drawer.	At the top.
Kick the ball.	Find the end.
At the back.	In the bag.
In the fridge.	On my own.
By myself.	By the door.
Ring the bell.	Halve the bill.
Take your time.	In the dark.
Climb the wall.	Catch a bus.
Fly a plane.	Ride a horse.
Ride a bike.	Hitch a lift.
Have a drink.	Cup of tea.
Glass of juice.	Lemon cake.
Glass of wine.	Hot crumpet.
Cold climate.	Bad tempered.
Good natured.	China cup.
Gleaming brass.	Yellow rose.
Narrow path.	Wide river.
Winter snow.	Autumn leaves.
Summer dress.	Spring fever.
Down below.	High above.
Write it down.	Make a note.
Take a rest.	Lovely day!
It's raining.	I'm hungry.
Let's go there.	Clap your hands.
Take cover!	Over there!
Buy these shoes.	Stretch your legs.

INTELLIGIBILITY 1 C

■ **Phrases/sentences with *four* syllables**

Over the door.
Under the chair.
In the garden.
A pinch of salt.
I'm fine, thank you.

Under the car.
On the table.
A new treatment.
Repeat that, please.
What time is it?

What do you think?
Milk and sugar?
Which road is it?
Read the letter.
Just the ticket.

Are you busy?
Supper's ready.
Find the number.
Renew a book.
Paint a picture.

Take the last bus.
Lose the paper.
Break a promise.
Write a letter.
Throw a party.

Buy a bargain.
Search the cupboard.
Read a novel.
Mind the baby.
Suck a toffee.

Watch the TV.
I'm feeling cold.
Come for coffee.
Sit in the sun.
Write up your notes.

Increase the sound.
I'm going home.
Turn right then left.
Look at that girl.
You're eating cake.

How do you feel?
May I come in?
Take care of Tom.
Look after Madge.
She's so clever.

You're looking well.
Of course you can.
The dog's all right.
Save your money.
Can you hear me?

What time is it?
His name is Dave.
Roses are red.

How old are you?
Swimming is fun.
He's very late.

C INTELLIGIBILITY 1

■ **Phrases/sentences with *five* syllables**

Return to London.
Say that again, please.
Please may I change this?
Is this seat taken?
In the hospital.

The kitchen is full.
Make a cup of tea.
Fill up with petrol.
Replace the lightbulb.
Practice makes perfect.

Are you pleased with it?
Can I go with you?
Open the bottle.
On your own again?
Behind the station.

Go on holiday.
Open for business.
Go out for a meal.
Book a holiday.
Is it ready now?

How long does it take?
Will you drive the car?
Watch the performance.
He just can't see it!
Play a game of chess.

INTELLIGIBILITY 1 C

■ **Phrases/sentences with *six* syllables**

To ski or not to ski?
Make room for the landlord.
Hand picked to pick the best.
How do you like it cooked?
Now take a drive in it.
Far from the madding crowd.
Expert or beginner?
Find the right place for it.
Give the dog his biscuit.
Underneath the table.
Let's see what they're doing.
She loves chocolate eclairs.
Give him another chance.
I'll write a cheque for that.

■ **Phrases/sentences with *seven* syllables**

Was this the one you wanted?
The beauty of a real fire.
Is this the best you can do?
Book a table for twenty.
Reserve the seats on the train.
Where is the best place to sit?
Will it take you all the way?
Don't get caught, get a licence.
Will you take a credit card?
We sent a bouquet of flowers.
Surely they're not going to Spain!
We fly non-stop to New York.

C INTELLIGIBILITY I

■ Longer than *seven*-syllable phrases/sentences

The shortest route to the station.
We'd like you to compare the two.
They can't complain about the service.
Let the experts pick up the pieces.
Arctic fishermen have the answer.
Composed from the finest ingredients.
Family fishing holidays in Sweden.
These days, children grow up in a fast-changing world.
This came about by design not by accident.
Is your oven as versatile as your cooking?

A reef knot is one of the simplest to learn how to tie.
I arrived in England ten years ago.
My mother's maiden name is Adamson.
Whisk eggs well before adding to sugar and butter.
Don't forget to use the Green Cross Code.
The early riser catches the worm.
Knit two together three times then cast off.
Please keep all medicine out of the reach of children.
Can you direct me to Piccadilly Circus?
Swimming is a most beneficial exercise.

INTELLIGIBILITY 1 C

■ **Longer than *seven*-syllable phrases/sentences**

There's nothing quite like gas for giving you control over your cooking.

Cheeses from Switzerland are pure delight for lovers of fine cheese everywhere.

Practical, nippy and economical, the new super-minis are hard to beat.

Valuable books should always be repaired by professionals.

Good lighting is an integral part of any fitted kitchen.

Its consumption of energy, water and detergent is amongst the lowest of any machine.

A holiday for two weeks in a luxurious Corfu villa for up to six people.

The robin isn't any common or garden bird.

How do you get more flavour from your baking?

Where did you put the washing powder and the washing-up liquid?

There is no allowance made for meals not taken.

Classic styles, in the best leathers, create a shoe that combines quality and comfort.

Traditionally created in long-established British factories.

My son Andrew came with me and was always a most helpful assistant.

It snowed all night long so by morning all the roads were impassable.

Before handling the samples please make sure that your hands are thoroughly clean.

SECTION 3
INTELLIGIBILITY II

This section contains a range of prose passages which may be used in a variety of ways. For example, they may be marked for:

- phrasing (long/short phrases);
- stress;
- final phoneme practice;
- specific type of phoneme practice (labials, velars, plosives and so on);
- consonant cluster practice.

The passages are grouped *approximately* according to reading level and complexity of language and/or articulatory difficulty. There are three levels suggested, each containing passages of increasing length and a variety of subject matter.

Rocking-chair

This traditional Boston rocking-chair is made from beechwood and is sanded, ready for polishing or painting. We have painted our rockers in red, white and blue to show how smart they look and you can paint yours in the colour of your choice or you may wish to leave it natural. The back and sides come fully assembled and the chairs are simple to put together. Full instructions, screws and glue are provided.

Wigmore Hall

Recognised from its earliest days as London's finest acoustic setting for chamber music, the Wigmore Hall has long been associated with concerts of French music. The tradition was firmly established during the war years, when a highly successful series of more than a hundred concerts of French music were given at the Wigmore Hall under Free French patronage.

Malta

The island of Malta is at the heart of the Mediterranean, set in crystal clear waters. Nothing is closer to the heart of the Maltese people than the happiness of her visitors. The reliable sunny climate, the richness of the island's history and the warm welcome extended to visitors have made this island a popular holiday destination. The island has a very British flavour with English spoken by almost everyone.

INTELLIGIBILITY II — Level I

Lindos

Lindos is one of the most famous villages in Greece. Shops, tavernas and bars cluster around the village square, and lovely whitewashed houses line the twisted, cobbled streets, too narrow for any car to pass. Set at the foot of a rocky headland, Lindos offers a unique combination of ancient history and modern activity. Many people return to Lindos year after year for its atmosphere.

The world is melting!

The ice fields and mountain snowcaps of the world are slowly melting. Sea level is rising about a millimetre every year, and many coastal cities will ultimately be flooded. A key element in this dire process is the creeping of ice fields and glaciers down from the heights where snowfall forms them, to lower, warmer regions where they melt.

Paint sample

Each small paint pot has its own brush and enough paint to cover a large piece of white card. By moving it around the room, you'll see what colour looks like under different lighting conditions. If you have a room that never sees the sun, you could paint it in a colour that captures the feeling of golden daffodils.

Leeds Castle

Surrounded by 500 acres of magnificent parkland and gardens, and built on two small islands in the middle of a natural lake, Leeds Castle is England's oldest and most romantic stately home. For some 300 years, the Castle was a favourite country palace of the Kings and Queens of medieval England.

Carrot and raisin salad

Peel the carrots, grate them coarsely and grind on lots of black pepper. If they are not to be used immediately, cover with film. Mix two teaspoons of salt with all the ground spices and the sugar and beat into the oil. When you are ready to finish the salad, drain the juices from the raisins into the spiced oil. Mix the raisins into the carrots and pour the oil over. Toss the salad thoroughly, then scatter with walnuts to garnish.

Yorkshire Terrier

Although the Yorkshire Terrier is one of the smallest breeds of dogs it has the courage and spirit of a brave guard dog. Yorkies, as they are popularly known, have fine, silky coats; steely blue on the upper body, and tan everywhere else. Although small, Yorkies enjoy a good walk and should be taken out at least once a day. Properly looked after, a Yorkie will be a faithful companion living well into its teens.

Low-cost flying

In the fiercely competitive world of aviation, the promise of a plane with lower operating costs than its rivals is driving aircraft manufacturers to spend millions of dollars on research. An obvious way to win the favour of airlines is to make planes that need less fuel. So engineers are designing planes which, for a given number of passengers and range, weigh less.

INTELLIGIBILITY II Level 2

Flower exhibition

The presentation of your exhibits can be most successful if a choice of colours is available in mixed classes, as careful placement of colours can greatly enhance an exhibit. In a close competition, the foliage is often the means by which awards are decided; so remove any spray residue and position the foliage to best advantage.

Planning a garden

I planned a sweeping border of roses for the front garden and employed two young men whom I had met in the village pub to double dig it for me, the manure coming from a nearby farm. It was a marathon work for the soil is heavy unyielding clay, blue and yellow. I intended planting potatoes to help break up the soil but my neighbours would not hear of this. They did not wish to look out on a potato patch! I had not had a garden of my own for nine years and was out of touch with the new rose varieties.

London

As the old music hall song says, this London is a wonderful place. So much to do, so much to see, you'll need to come back again and again. There's historic London with its palaces and fortifications, its churches and houses, in which once lived the famous and the infamous. There's fashionable London with its elegant streets and beautiful squares. There's a London to delight the ladies, with fine shops and boutiques. A London of museums and art galleries for the curious. A London of light and bustle where theatre and cinema neon beckons. There's the London of today, with its red buses, black cabs, friendly bobbies and everywhere the hustle, bustle and fun of a great city. Ah! London . . . when you're tired of London you're tired of life.

National Garden Festival

Set in 180 acres, the National Garden Festival offers so much to see and enjoy. There are eighty fabulous theme gardens; three lakes with bridges, cascades and glorious landscapes; over fifty continuous horticultural shows in the Festival Hall; one hundred and fifty stalls from pottery to pot plants; thousands of events such as hot air balloons, clowns, stilt men, massed bands, jazz groups, theatre shows, boat rallies and much, much more. There are ten super show homes with prize-winning gardens. More than 250,000 trees, millions of plants, shrubs and flowers. Choose from a variety of places to eat and drink or, if you prefer, picnic on one of the many grassy banks. Enjoy the panoramic view from a cable car or travel around on one of the festival trains.

Children's World

Boots the chemist has for many years been one of the High Street's leading retailers of products for babies and young children, and your local stores will continue to provide the high standards of service Boots customers expect. The Boots company now also invites you to an exciting shopping experience at our new edge-of-town children's superstore, Children's World. Whether you are a parent, parent-to-be or just buying for children, Children's World has been created to make shopping a more enjoyable experience for all our customers, large and small.

Guaranteed Waterproof!

If you've been searching for a really comfortable but genuine waterproof and weather beating pair of storm boots, look no further. These newly designed boots are made to the highest standards which guarantee that no matter how bad the weather conditions underfoot in town or country you will be kept warm, dry and completely comfortable. The combination of strength and lightness make them suitable not just for winter wear but also for stormy weather throughout the year.

INTELLIGIBILITY II Level 2

Yorkshire

Come and discover some of the largest tracts of unspoilt countryside in England. To the west of the region stands the Pennine range — the 'Backbone of England' — and superb walking country. From these rugged hills and mountains descend the famous Yorkshire Dales, vast expanses of moorland, fast-flowing rivers, plunging waterfalls and wooded gorges. Contrast spectacular scenery like this with the gentler beauty of the Vale of York, a broad lowland expanse, woven through with great rivers. In the Vale of York, you must visit York Minster — its medieval stained glass windows are among the art treasures of the world.

Hong Kong

In Hong Kong, choosing a name is a serious matter because of the ancient belief that what you are called is what you will become. That's why, ever since the book about the famous Hong Kong bar-girl came out, the Wongs have avoided the name Suzie. Mysticism and modern living go hand in hand in Hong Kong. They are part of the way of life which makes this unique city so fascinating — a place where the unusual is ordinary and the extraordinary is commonplace.

Holidays

Yugoslavia has one of the most magnificent coasts in Europe. In the north, the Venetian influence is apparent in many of the towns and cities of the Istrian coast. In the south, the Dalmatian Coast stretches along the Adriatic against a background of terraced vineyards. Here the medieval city of Dubrovnik mingles with modern holiday resorts and small islands of great beauty.

Level 2 INTELLIGIBILITY II

Dining out in Greece

Dining in one of the many tavernas is an essential and enjoyable part of your holiday. They are small, friendly and offer good variety and exceptional value. As well as the famous kebabs, try the delicious grilled seafood — often you are invited to go into the kitchen to choose your own fish! Local wines and lager beer are inexpensive. Dinner for two can cost as little as £6.

Yugoslavia

For the holidaymaker, Yugoslavia offers exceptional value. Whatever you seek, Yugoslavia will provide it in abundance. If you want sun, then Europe's most glorious coastline can scarcely disappoint. If you enjoy walking or sightseeing, the richly varied landscape and historic towns will captivate your imagination. But not only is this beautiful country blessed with natural and cultural riches, one of its greatest assets is its people. Warm and courteous and fiercely proud of their country, the Yugoslavs will do all they can to ensure that you enjoy your stay. Limestone hills, often thickly wooded, spill down into the deep blue of the Adriatic to form this spectacularly beautiful coastline. With the sea penetrating far inland, attractive coves and bays are to be found everywhere. Although not many are of sand, the beaches are ideal for bathing, for nearly all are gently sloping and shallow.

INTELLIGIBILITY II Level 2

The Royal Naval College, Greenwich

The College stands on the site of the Royal Palace of Greenwich, the main seat of Tudor monarchs and the birthplace of Henry VII, Mary I and Elizabeth I. Wren was commissioned to build the College when the site of the Palace was donated by William and Mary for the purpose of a naval hospital similar to the Army Hospital at Chelsea. Greenwich Hospital, as it was then known, was used as a naval hospital housing almost 3,000 Pensioners until 1869. In 1873 the Admiralty took over the building for educational purposes and the College now acts as the Royal Navy's University. The Chapel, which is dedicated to St Peter and St Paul, has a dome and a colonnade which are unmistakably Wren, but the baroque interior originally designed by Wren and Ripley was gutted by fire in 1779.

Southampton

Southampton has been one of Britain's major gateways since the Romans established a port on the River Itchen. During the Middle Ages the city was fortified and much remains of the impressive walls and gateways. Most people connect Southampton with ships and docks but the city has much more to offer, combining a busy commercial centre with the rural beauty of Southern England. The city offers all the amenities the visitor would expect to find, plenty of entertainment venues and a host of interesting places to visit in the surrounding area.

Salisbury

Salisbury is an attractive market city dominated by the magnificent cathedral with its 404 feet high spire. The Cathedral Close is the largest in Britain and contains two museums. The prehistoric stone circle of Stonehenge stands in bleak surroundings on Salisbury Plain. Its origins go back to 2800BC; some of the stones were transported from the Prescelly Mountains in Wales. The Druids hold a ceremony annually at sunrise on Midsummer morning.

Level 2 INTELLIGIBILITY II

Wine

Here's your chance to discover what's really behind the label when you buy a bottle of French wine. You'll find out why wines taste different and why some bottles cost more than others! Come, glass in hand, on an armchair tour of France, as we taste our way through the wine regions from Bordeaux to Champagne. Did you know that wine has been made in England since vines were first planted by the Romans 2,000 years ago? We'll be visiting the successful Three Choirs vineyard, among the largest in Britain, for a guided tour and tasting. Throw away the textbooks and see what happens in a real commercial vineyard.

Museum of Mankind

The Museum of Mankind presents a series of changing exhibitions which illustrate the variety of non-Western societies and cultures. The Museum's collections come from the indigenous peoples of Africa, Australia and the Pacific Islands, North and South Africa and from certain parts of Asia and Europe, including some ancient as well as recent and contemporary cultures. Exhibitions depict the way of life of particular people or focus on specific aspects of their cultures.

Garden and the law

This is a great time of year to start planning a garden and, as far as I know, no one can ever stop you from growing whatever type of flowers you like, but what you do with your hedges, trees, garden sheds and so on is another matter. I'm assured by local authorities that the principle of planning regulations is to allow you to do as you please with your gardens, unless it interferes with others. Hedges, in fact, are of no interest to local authorities at all, unless they are beside a public right of way. If they are, make sure that they aren't sticking into the road or over the pavement, because if one of your neighbours is poked in the eye by a hawthorn twig, there could be trouble.

INTELLIGIBILITY II Level 2

Laura Ashley

Some people seem to believe that everything designed by Laura Ashley is festooned with flowers. Not quite true, though our love of flowers has not wilted. Our shops are still blooming but they are also full of bold stripes, checks, Paisley, shells and trellises — as well as more abstract patterns and plain co-ordinating colours. Whether our fabrics and wallpapers feature roses or rhomboids, they are all based on traditional designs chosen for their timeless elegance.

Rhodes

Rhodes is certainly one of the most beautiful Greek islands, with a profusion of bright flowers, lush valleys and inviting beaches. The island is steeped in history, with many magnificent monuments still remaining as a reminder of Rhodes' past. The old town is charming, with medieval houses and palaces hidden among narrow, cobbled streets. In contrast the new town has been transformed, owing to largely Italian influence, into a cosmopolitan and sophisticated centre.

Vintage Cars

Just imagine if the next time you popped out to the shops in your car, you had to get a man to walk in front of you carrying a red flag. And how about being fined for speeding more than 10 miles an hour, or trying to reach the nearest garage, 50 miles away, with no guarantee of there being any petrol available when you got there? The newly invented automobile was first seen purely as a plaything for the very rich — few could have dreamed that one day millions of people would own a car of their own. Go back less than 90 years to the beginning of the Edwardian era and motoring was still a very risky venture indeed.

Level 3 INTELLIGIBILITY II

Distinctive Inns

Have you ever longed to escape to a secluded country cottage, or take high tea on the lawns of an English country Manor House? Or would you like to make a pilgrimage to a twelfth-century Benedictine Monastery and rest overnight at England's oldest inn? Or spend a day fishing on a lake in the grounds of a Royal Palace before retiring to an historic coaching inn?

The distinctive inns, situated in the peaceful English countryside of the Cotswolds, Berkshire and Sussex, create idyllic settings for a very special break. These historic hotels all retain their traditional charm and character, yet have been tastefully modernised to suit today's visitor. All the inns hold a very high reputation for their excellent food and superb accommodation which, combined with a warmth of service, will ensure that you will enjoy a truly traditional English weekend.

Amsterdam

Amsterdam is a fascinating place of contradictions. It is an undeniably rich city, yet the most popular drinking places are called 'brown bars', loved for the very sparseness of the décor. Amsterdam's people are the greatest contradiction of all. While they are generally industrious, sober-minded and domestically inclined, their city is filled with shops, restaurants, artistic distractions of the highest calibre and raucous entertainment that shocks, yet certainly manages to intrigue.

This England

Many different themes combine to form the landscape of the Heart of England. The flat patchwork of Norfolk and the gleaming Broads contrast with the craggy North Derbyshire Peak District. Compare the peaceful sheep-nibbled uplands of Northamptonshire and Leicestershire with the bustling energy of Birmingham, Britain's second largest city. In an area offering such tremendous variety, you are spoiled for choice. Explore the broad river valley and gentle green countryside around Shakespeare's Stratford-upon-Avon and nearby Cotswold Hills. Discover magnificent Cannock Chase, miles of protected moorland and forest, which was once a Royal hunting-ground. Wander over the rolling chalk uplands of the Leicestershire wolds, with their quiet streams and beautiful hanging beechwoods. Wherever you choose to stay, you will find areas of outstanding scenic beauty within motoring distance.

Early Music

What is 'Early Music'? It now seems to encompass everything from plainsong to fortepianos, and this new South Bank series of concerts stretches from the medieval secular extravaganza of the New London Consort and the pilgrimage songs of the Martin Best Ensemble all the way to Beethoven symphonies played on period instruments by the London Classical Players.

What links the work of all the groups represented in this series — which aims to present a 'state of the art' collection of the best work across the whole field of early music — is a refusal to accept performance traditions as they have developed over the last century or two, and a determination to return to period style, using period instruments and every scrap of information that can be gleaned from written information, in order to animate their modern performances.

The Academy of St Martin-in-the Fields

Since its modest beginning giving a series of recitals in St Martin-in-the-Fields during a foggy November in 1959, the Academy of St Martin-in-the-Fields has gained an international reputation second to none as one of the finest and most versatile ensembles in the world. The name of the Academy has spread far and wide as a synonym for excellence through its several hundred recordings and many overseas concert performances undertaken every year. From an original basic ensemble of sixteen string players, the Academy has grown and matured into a constituent ensemble that can successfully perform a repertoire requiring anything from seven to seventy players.

Roses

The blooms of large-flowered roses should be protected from adverse weather by covering the selected buds when the calyx first opens to reveal petal colour. This protection may be by the conventional shade attached to a stick. Owing to the difficulty in obtaining these, a polythene bag secured by a wire twist may be an alternative. To combat condensation, a small half circle hole cut into each side of the bag will allow extra air to circulate. These bags may be used in conjunction with the shades to give extra protection in windy conditions, and an additional stake to secure the flower-bearing stem is an extra precaution.

Royal National Rose Society

May is a very critical month for the timing of roses for exhibition; a fortnight of cold, dry weather at this time will seriously affect all your expectations by retarding what might have appeared to be a most promising start to the season. All your efforts should be directed into promoting good, steady growth; forced growth will often result in small flowers and weak foot-stalks. Watering can be beneficial in periods of drought. However, do ensure that the soil is well moistened; too little water may prove detrimental. Any application of chemical fertiliser should be undertaken when the soil is moist. When spraying pesticides and foliar feeds, care should be taken that these do not fall on the developing flower buds, as they can cause damage.

Natural health

There is rarely one isolated factor as the cause of an illness or disease. The pain or symptom experienced is often a final manifestation of a long, gradual and complex process. The treatments offered all aim to treat the causes of ill-health in a balanced way. A priority, however, will always be to alleviate pain and make the patient feel comfortable. These treatments need not conflict in any way with orthodox medical treatment. They not only combat disease but create a pattern for health and the prevention of future illness.

Biofeedback

By making a person aware of the natural biofeedback systems which are operating within the body, the instruments allow the individual to exert a certain amount of control over these internal functions. He can try to change them by altering his subjective or behavioural states, usually by some form of relaxation or meditation. Any change he is able to bring about is immediately known to him through the display system. By trial and error, as well as through the therapist's guidance, he can learn to control a particular function. The idea behind the procedure is that the knowledge of success reinforces the learning; in other words, success breeds success.

Rudolf Steiner Education

Rudolf Steiner Education is concerned equally with the development of thinking, feeling and willing, the three basic faculties of human experience. In the Kindergarten, the main emphasis is on the education of the will — the impulse to do things. In the Lower School, the emphasis shifts to the education of the heart — the imaginative and emotional life. In the Upper School, the accent is on the education of thinking and the development of personal judgement. The curriculum recognises the inner needs of the child at different stages of development, not only with changes in the style and method of teaching, but also with careful choices of teaching material.

Photography

We can all take these pictures, the ones that give such a pleasurable return. You don't need elaborate, expensive equipment with which to make a start, so don't rush out to your nearest photographic dealer, breathlessly demanding to see the very latest developments in electronic and photographic machinery. Whatever camera you have at the moment, you can observe certain basic rules and take some excellent pictures. Later on we can look at interchangeable lenses, exposure times, macro-converters, f-numbers and all the mystic things which give you more flexibility but which are not essential.

The Hedgehog

We generally think of the hedgehog as being a countryside animal, but it is becoming increasingly common in British towns and cities. As its name suggests, the hedgehog makes its home in dry grass and leaves under our hedgerows. But even in a neglected corner of a park or garden a hedgehog may still find a cosy place to make its nest. Since the animals are nocturnal you stand a better chance of seeing one at night. The hedgehog eats beetles, caterpillars and earthworms, but if you are hoping to attract one to your garden, a saucer of bread and milk is a tempting treat. The hedgehog has few enemies, thanks to its protective coat of spines. When threatened, it curls up into a tight, prickly ball. The young who have fewer spines or haven't learned to curl up properly sometimes fall prey to predators such as foxes. The hedgehog is at greatest risk during winter hibernation. It is estimated that more than half the hedgehog population does not survive its first winter.

SECTION 4
PROSODY I

This section concentrates on **stress** and provides a wide range of exercises for within-word stress. There is also a series of contrastive stress drill dialogues and, finally, a range of limericks and poems for rhythmic word/syllable stress practice.

A	**Syllable stress changes according to word class**	85
B	**Contrastive stress drills**	91
C	**Limericks**	97
D	**Poems**	99

Syllable stress changes according to word class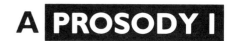

conduct (noun)
Parents expect good **con**duct from their children.
Con**duct** (verb)
Andre Previn will con**duct** the orchestra tonight.

record (noun)
Ed Moses holds the **re**cord for the 100 metres.
re**cord** (verb)
Some people re**cord** daily events in a diary.

present (noun, adjective)
Her birthday **pre**sent was a complete surprise.
At the **pre**sent time we have three applicants for the job.
pre**sent** (verb)
My daughter will pre**sent** a bouquet to the Queen.

dictate (noun)
The **dic**tate prevents us leaving the country without a permit.
dic**tate** (verb)
Please dic**tate** the letter more slowly.

convert (noun)
He was a **con**vert to Buddhist beliefs.
con**vert** (verb)
We plan to con**vert** the barn into a large house.

upset (noun)
The loss of her ring was a great **up**set.
up**set** (verb, adjective)
The boisterous dog up**set** the vase of flowers.
The little girl was up**set** when she fell over.

transfer (noun)
He wanted a **trans**fer to another department.
trans**fer** (verb)
I will trans**fer** the money to my current account.

transport (noun)
Cars, buses and boats are all forms of **trans**port.
trans**port** (verb)
Can you trans**port** these goods to London by Friday?

PROSODY 1 A

produce (noun)
They sell **pro**duce of the best quality.
pro**duce** (verb)
To pro**duce** a play well requires co-operation from all involved.

conflict (verb)
The **con**flict between the two men was brief but decisive.
con**flict** (verb)
These appointments con**flict** with other arrangements.

contract (noun)
The terms of the **con**tract are legal and binding.
con**tract** (verb)
Our pupils con**tract** in bright light.

contrast (noun)
There is a clear **con**trast between black and white.
con**trast** (verb)
You must con**trast** one dress with another when making your choice.

converse (noun)
What you say now is the **con**verse of your earlier ideas.
con**verse** (verb)
Can you con**verse** in French?

contest (noun)
The **con**test was between two well-matched opponents.
con**test** (verb)
You may con**test** the will if you think it is unfair.

convict (noun)
The **con**victs were transported to Australia.
con**vict** (verb)
The jury must con**vict** him of murder.

combine (noun)
It was a **com**bine of several companies.
com**bine** (verb)
The two businesses must com**bine** to succeed.

A PROSODY 1

compress (noun)
Apply a cold **com**press to your swollen ankle.
com**press** (verb)
Old cars are com**press**ed for scrap metal.

conscript (noun)
He joined the army as a **con**script.
con**script** (verb)
We no longer con**script** men into the armed forces.

concert (noun)
Most people enjoy a good **con**cert.
con**cert** (verb)
We must con**cert** our efforts to complete the job.

console (noun)
He sat alone at the organ **con**sole.
con**sole** (verb)
She tried to con**sole** the family who had been robbed.

compact (noun)
She kept her powder in a pretty **com**pact.
com**pact** (adjective)
The gymnast's build is com**pact**.

absent (adjective)
She was **ab**sent from work all week.
ab**sent** (verb)
Don't ab**sent** yourself when you are needed.

abstract (noun)
Here is an **ab**stract from his speech.
ab**stract** (verb)
You must ab**stract** the information you find useful.

attribute (noun)
Punctuality is his main **at**tribute.
at**tribu**te (verb)
He can at**tribu**te his success to sheer hard work.

PROSODY I A

accent (noun)
We know by his **ac**cent that he is Welsh.
ac**cent** (verb)
You should ac**cent** the second syllable in this word.

addict (noun)
Too many young people are drug **ad**dicts.
ad**dict** (verb)
Do not become ad**dict**ed to drugs.

decrease (noun)
There is a current **de**crease in Britain's population.
de**crease** (verb)
The number of new students continues to de**crease**.

desert (noun)
The camel is the 'ship of the **de**sert'.
de**sert** (verb)
You must not de**sert** anyone in need.

digest (noun)
*Readers' **Di**gest* is a popular magazine.
di**gest** (verb)
Allow enough time to di**gest** your food.

impact (noun)
The cars collided with an immense **im**pact.
im**pact** (verb)
The tooth is im**pact**ed in his jaw.

implant (noun)
The balding man asked for an **im**plant of new hair.
im**plant** (verb)
It is now possible to im**plant** a pacemaker in the body.

increase (noun)
There has been a recent **in**crease in violent crime.
in**crease** (verb)
Knitters must be able to in**crease** the number of stitches on their needles.

A PROSODY I

object (noun)
The artefact was an **ob**ject of great interest.
ob**ject** (verb)
Do you ob**ject** to these suggestions?

pervert (noun)
The convicted criminal was a **per**vert.
per**vert** (verb)
Do not try to per**vert** the course of justice.

rebel (noun)
Was James Dean a **re**bel without a cause?
re**bel** (verb)
Most children re**bel** about going to school.

rebound (noun)
He caught the ball on the **re**bound.
re**bound** (verb)
His behaviour may re**bound** on him later.

refuse (noun)
Refuse must be cleared regularly.
re**fuse** (verb)
Do you re**fuse** to obey?

reject (noun)
The cracked cup was a **re**ject.
re**ject** (verb)
Unfortunately we must re**ject** his application.

subject (noun)
What is the **sub**ject of the plot?
sub**ject** (verb)
Must you sub**ject** her to so many tests?

second (adjective, verb)
Mary came **se**cond in the race.
Will anyone **se**cond my proposal?
se**cond** (verb)
They may se**cond** you to another branch.

PROSODY I A

suspect (noun)
The prime **sus**pect is missing.
sus**pect** (verb)
What do you sus**pect** him of?

permit (noun)
Do you have a fishing **per**mit?
per**mit** (verb)
Will you per**mit** me to leave?

construct (noun)
This is a hard **con**struct to grasp.
con**struct** (verb)
You must con**struct** a bigger shed.

Contrastive stress drills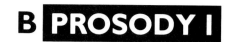

■ **Short sentences with monosyllabic words**

Therapist

Wild dogs eat meat.
Which dogs eat meat?
Do wild **cats** eat meat?
Do wild dogs **hunt** meat?
Do wild dogs eat **grass**?

All cows eat grass.
Do **some** cows eat grass?
Do all **pigs** eat grass?
Do all cows **cut** grass?
Do all cows eat **cheese**?

Red cars look smart.
Which cars look smart?
Do red **vans** look smart?
Do red cars look **scruffy**?

My coat is blue.
Whose coat is blue?
Is **his** coat blue?
Is your **hat** blue?
Is your coat **grey**?

His name is Paul.
Whose name is Paul?
His name's **not** Paul.
Is his name **John**?

That bag feels light.
Which bag feels light?
Does that **box** feel light?
Does that bag **look** light?
Does that bag feel **heavy**?

Patient

Wild dogs eat meat.
Wild dogs eat meat.
No, wild **dogs** eat meat.
No, wild dogs **eat** meat.
No, wild dogs eat **meat**.

All cows eat grass.
No, **all** cows eat grass.
No, all **cows** eat grass.
No, all cows **eat** grass.
No, all cows eat **grass**.

Red cars look smart.
Red cars look smart.
No, red **cars** look smart.
No, red cars look **smart**.

My coat is blue.
My coat is blue.
No, **my** coat is blue.
No, my **coat** is blue.
No, my coat is **blue**.

His name is Paul.
His name is Paul.
His name **is** Paul.
No, his name is **Paul**.

That bag feels light.
That bag feels light.
No, that **bag** feels light.
No, that bag **feels** light.
No, that bag feels **light**.

PROSODY 1 B

Therapist	*Patient*

I want four stamps.
Who wants four stamps?
Do you **need** four stamps?
Do you want **three** stamps?
Do you want four **pens**?

Small boys like sweets.
Which boys like sweets?
Do small **girls** like sweets?
Do small boys **hate** sweets?
Do small boys like **snails**?

Sue cuts Dave's hair.
Who cuts Dave's hair?
Does Sue **comb** Dave's hair?
Does Sue cut **John's** hair?
Does Sue cut Dave's **nails**?

May bakes fruit pies.
Who bakes fruit pies?
Does May **eat** fruit pies?
Does May bake **meat** pies?
Does May bake fruit **cake**?

Most men work hard.
Do **all** men work hard?
Do most **boys** work hard?
Do most men **look** hard?
Do most men work **slowly**?

This shop sells books.
Which shop sells books?
Does this **house** sell books?
Does this shop **buy** books?
Does this shop sell **pens**?

I want four stamps.
I want four stamps.
I **want** four stamps.
No, I want **four** stamps.
No, I want four **stamps**.

Small boys like sweets.
Small boys like sweets.
No, small **boys** like sweets.
No, small boys **like** sweets.
No, small boys like **sweets**.

Sue cuts Dave's hair.
Sue cuts Dave's hair.
No, Sue **cuts** Dave's hair.
No, Sue cuts **Dave's** hair.
No, Sue cuts Dave's **hair**.

May bakes fruit pies.
May bakes fruit pies.
No, May **bakes** fruit pies.
No, May bakes **fruit** pies.
No, May bakes fruit **pies**.

Most men work hard.
Most men work hard.
No, most **men** work hard.
No, most men **work** hard.
No, most men work **hard**.

This shop sells books.
This shop sells books.
No, this **shop** sells books.
No, this shop **sells** books.
No, this ship sells **books**.

B PROSODY 1

Therapist	*Patient*
Some girls wear pink.	Some girls wear pink.
Do **all** girls wear pink?	No, **some** girls wear pink.
Do some **boys** wear pink?	No, some **girls** wear pink.
Do some girls **like** pink?	No, some girls **wear** pink.
Do some girls wear **green**?	No, some girls wear **pink**.
My feet are cold.	My feet are cold.
Whose feet are cold?	**My** feet are cold.
Are your **hands** cold?	No, my **feet** are cold.
Your feet **aren't** cold.	My feet **are** cold.
Are your feet **hot**?	No, my feet are **cold**.
Eve's hands are clean.	Eve's hands are clean.
Whose hands are clean?	**Eve's** hands are clean.
Are Eve's **ears** clean?	No, Eve's **hands** are clean.
Eve's hands **aren't** clean.	Eve's hands **are** clean.
Are Eve's hands **dirty**?	No, Eve's hands are **clean**.
John wore a red jumper.	John wore a red jumper.
Who wore a red jumper?	**John** wore a red jumper.
Did John wear a **blue** jumper?	No, John wore a **red** jumper.
Did John **wash** a red jumper?	No, John **wore** a red jumper.
Did John wear a red **scarf**?	No, John wore a red **jumper**.
Dave bought a new car.	Dave bought a new car.
Who bought a new car?	**Dave** bought a new car.
Did Dave buy a new **bicycle**?	No, Dave bought a new **car**.
Did Dave **hire** a new car?	No, Dave **bought** a new car.
Did Dave buy a **second-hand** car?	No, Dave bought a **new** car.

PROSODY I B

■ Short sentences with bisyllabic words

Therapist

Nick caught the train at six o'clock.
Who caught the train at six o'clock?
Did Nick catch the train at **five** o'clock?
Did Nick catch the **bus** at six o'clock?
Did Nick **miss** the train at six o'clock?

Simon is Betty's nephew.
Who is Betty's nephew?
Simon is **not** Betty's nephew.
Is Simon Betty's **niece**?
Is Simon **your** nephew?

Red balloons are nicest.
Are **blue** balloons nicest?
Are red **ribbons** nicest?
Are red balloons **smallest**?

Dave plays the trombone very well.
Who plays the trombone very well?
Does Dave play the **banjo** very well?
Does Dave play the trombone **quite** well?
Does Dave play the trombone very **badly**?
Does Dave **hear** the trombone very well?

Patient

Nick caught the train at six o'clock.
Nick caught the train at six o'clock.
No, Nick caught the train at **six** o'clock.
No, Nick caught the **train** at six o'clock.
No, Nick **caught** the train at six o'clock.

Simon is Betty's nephew.
Simon is Betty's nephew.
Simon **is** Betty's nephew.
No, Simon is Betty's **nephew**.
No, Simon is **Betty's** nephew.

Red balloons are nicest.
No **red** balloons are nicest.
No, red **balloons** are nicest.
No, red balloons are **nicest**.

Dave plays the trombone very well.
Dave plays the trombone very well.
No, Dave plays the **trombone** very well.
No, Dave plays the trombone **very** well.
No, Dave plays the trombone very **well**.
No, Dave **plays** the trombone very well.

B PROSODY I

Therapist	Patient
The plumber will come tomorrow at two.	The plumber will come tomorrow at two.
When will the plumber come?	The plumber will come **tomorrow at two**.
Will the plumber come **today** at two?	No, the plumber will come **tomorrow** at two.
Will he come tomorrow at **three**?	No, he will come tomorrow at **two**.
Who will come tomorrow at two?	The **plumber** will come tomorrow at two.
Will the plumber **leave** tomorrow at two?	No, the plumber will **come** tomorrow at two.
Val drives a large white van.	Val drives a large white van.
Who drives a large white van?	**Val** drives a large white van.
Does Val drive a **small** white van?	No, Val drives a **large** white van.
Does Val drive a large white **bus**?	No, Val drives a large white **van**.
Does Val **buy** a large white van?	No, Val **drives** a large white van.
Basil is wearing a checked hat.	Basil is wearing a checked hat.
Who is wearing a checked hat?	**Basil** is wearing a checked hat.
Is Basil **carrying** a checked hat?	No, Basil is **wearing** a checked hat.
Is Basil wearing a **striped** hat?	No, Basil is wearing a **checked** hat.
Is Basil wearing a checked **suit**?	No, Basil is wearing a checked **hat**.
Is **Tom** wearing a checked hat?	No, **Basil** is wearing a checked hat.
There are twelve months in every year.	There are twelve months in every year.
Are there **ten** months in every year?	No, there are **twelve** months in every year.
Are there twelve **weeks** in every year?	No, there are twelve **months** in every year.
Are there twelve months in **some** years?	No, there are twelve months in **every** year.
Are there twelve months in every **season**?	No, there are twelve months in every **year**.

PROSODY I B

Therapist	*Patient*
Steve was the fastest runner in the mile.	Steve was the fastest runner in the mile.
Who was the fastest runner in the mile?	**Steve** was the fastest runner in the mile.
Was Steve the **slowest** runner in the mile?	No, Steve was the **fastest** runner in the mile.
Was Steve the fastest **walker** in the mile?	No, Steve was the fastest **runner** in the mile.
Was Steve the fastest runner in the **sprint**?	No, Steve was the fastest runner in the **mile**.
The lion is the king of the jungle.	The lion is the king of the jungle.
Who is the king of the jungle?	The **lion** is the king of the jungle.
Is the lion the **master** of the jungle?	No, the lion is the **king** of the jungle.
Is the lion the king of the **sea**?	No, the lion is the king of the **jungle**.
His friend is a good driver.	His friend is a good driver.
Whose friend is a good driver?	**His** friend is a good driver.
Is **he** a good driver?	No, his **friend** is a good driver.
Is his friend a **bad** driver?	No, his friend is a **good** driver.
Is his friend a good **runner**?	No, his friend is a good **driver**.
That girl never listens to advice.	That girl never listens to advice.
Which girl never listens to advice?	**That** girl never listens to advice.
Does that girl **ever** listen to advice?	No, that girl **never** listens to advice.
Does that **boy** never listen to advice?	No, that **girl** never listens to advice.
Does that girl never listen to **music**?	No, that girl never listens to **advice**.
Does that girl never **offer** advice?	No, that girl never **listens** to advice.

Limericks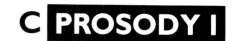

There was an Old Person of Cheadle,
Was put in the stocks by the beadle;
    For stealing some pigs,
    Some coats and some wigs,
That horrible Person of Cheadle.

There was an Old Man of Dundee,
Who frequented the top of a tree;
    When disturbed by the crows,
    He abruptly arose,
And exclaimed, "I'll return to Dundee."

There was a Young Lady of Norway,
Who casually sat in a doorway;
    When the door squeezed her flat,
    She exclaimed, "What of that?"
This courageous Young Lady of Norway.

Edward Lear

There was an old Fellow of Trinity,
A Doctor well versed in Divinity,
    But he took to free thinking
    And then to deep drinking,
And so had to leave the vicinity.

Arthur Clement Hilton

PROSODY 1 C

There was a young lady named Bright
Whose speed was far faster than light.
     She set out one day
     In a relative way,
And returned home the previous night.

Arthur Buller

A wonderful bird is the pelican;
His bill can hold more than his belican.
     He can take in his beak
     Food enough for a week;
But I'm damned if I see how the helican!

Dixon Lanier Merritt

There was a young lady of Ryde
Who ate a green apple and died;
     The apple fermented
     Inside the lamented,
And made cider inside her inside.

There was an old man of Peru,
Who dreamt he was eating his shoe.
     He woke in the night
     In a terrible fright,
And found it was perfectly true.

Punch

Do You Have It In A 60 Extra-Long?

To me it's inconceivable
That one could find believable
The thought that one must have a shape
Exactly like his chum.
I simply won't apologise
For being a grander size —
When everyone's a seedless grape
It's great to be a plum.

Victor Buono

The Rum Tum Tugger

The Rum Tum Tugger is a Curious Cat:
If you offer him pheasant he would rather have grouse.
If you put him in a house he would much prefer a flat,
If you put him in a flat then he'd rather have a house.
If you set him on a mouse then he only wants a rat,
If you set him on a rat then he'd rather chase a mouse.
Yes the Rum Tum Tugger is a Curious Cat—
   And there isn't any call for me to shout it:
      For he will do
      As he do do
         And there's no doing anything about it!

The Rum Tum Tugger is a terrible bore:
When you let him in, then he wants to be out;
He's always on the wrong side of every door,
And as soon as he's at home, then he'd like to get about.
He likes to lie in the bureau drawer,
But he makes such a fuss if he can't get out.
Yes the Rum Tum Tugger is a Curious Cat—
   And it isn't any use for you to doubt it:
      For he will do
      As he do do
         And there's no doing anything about it!

PROSODY I D

The Rum Tum Tugger is a curious beast:
His disobliging ways are a matter of habit.
If you offer him fish then he always wants a feast;
When there isn't any fish then he won't eat rabbit.
If you offer him cream then he sniffs and sneers,
For he only likes what he finds for himself;
So you'll catch him in it right up to the ears,
If you put it away on the larder shelf.
The Rum Tum Tugger is artful and knowing,
The Rum Tum Tugger doesn't care for a cuddle;
But he'll leap on your lap in the middle of your sewing,
For there's nothing he enjoys like a horrible muddle.
Yes the Rum Tum Tugger is a Curious Cat—
    And there isn't any need for me to spout it:
        For he will do
        As he do do
            And there's no doing anything about it!

TS Eliot

A Fat Man's Prayer

Lord my soul is ripped with riot
Incited by my wicked diet;
"We are what we eat" said a wise old man,
And Lord if that's true, I'm a garbage can.

To rise on Judgement Day it's plain
That at my weight I'll need a crane,
So grant me strength that I may not fall
Into the clutches of cholesterol.

Victor Buono

You Are Old, Father William

"You are old, Father William," the young man said.
    "And your hair has become very white;
And yet you incessantly stand on your head —
    Do you think, at your age, it is right?"

"In my youth," Father William replied to his son,
    "I feared it might injure the brain;
But, now that I'm perfectly sure I have none,
    Why, I do it again and again."

Lewis Carroll

PROSODY I D

Daffodils

I wandered lonely as a cloud
     That floats on high o'er vales and hills,
When all at once I saw a crowd,
     A host of golden daffodils;
Beside the lake, beneath the trees,
Fluttering and dancing in the breeze.

Continuous as the stars that shine
     And twinkle on the Milky Way,
They stretched in never-ending line
     Along the margin of a bay:
Ten thousand saw I at a glance,
Tossing their heads in sprightly dance.

William Wordsworth

Lochinvar

O, young Lochinvar is come out of the west,
Through all the wide Border his steed was the best;
And save his good broadsword he weapons had none,
He rode all unarm'd, and he rode all alone.
So faithful in love, and so dauntless in war,
There never was knight like the young Lochinvar.

Sir Walter Scott

Cargoes

Dirty British coaster with a salt-caked smoke stack
Butting through the Channel in the mad March days,
With a cargo of Tyne coal,
Road-rail, pig-lead,
Firewood, iron-ware, and cheap tin trays.

John Masefield

Sea-Fever

I must down to the seas again, to the lonely sea and the sky,
And all I ask is a tall ship and a star to steer her by,
And the wheel's kick and the wind's song and the white sails shaking,
And a grey mist on the sea's face and a grey dawn breaking.

I must down to the seas again, for the call of the running tide
Is a wild call and a clear call that may not be denied;
And all I ask is a windy day with the white clouds flying,
And the flung spray and the blown spume, and the sea-gulls crying.

I must down to the seas again, to the vagrant gypsy life,
To the gull's way and the whale's way where the wind's like a whetted knife;
And all I ask is a merry yarn from a laughing fellow-rover,
And quiet sleep and a sweet dream when the long trick's over.

John Masefield

PROSODY I D

Night Mail

(Commentary for a GPO Film)

I

This is the Night Mail crossing the Border,
Bringing the cheque and the postal order,

Letters for the rich, letters for the poor,
The shop at the corner, the girl next door.

Pulling up Beattock, a steady climb:
The gradient's against her, but she's on time.

Past cotton-grass and moorland boulder,
Shovelling white steam over her shoulder,

Snorting noisily, she passes
Silent miles of wind-bent grasses.

III

Letters of thanks, letters from banks,
Letters of joy from girl and boy,
Receipted bills and invitations
To inspect new stock or to visit relations,
And applications for situations,
And timid lovers' declarations,
And gossip, gossip from all the nations,
News circumstantial, news financial,
Letters with holiday snaps to enlarge in,
Letters with faces scrawled on the margin,
Letters from uncles, cousins and aunts,
Letters to Scotland from the South of France,
Letters of condolence to Highlands and Lowlands,
Written on paper of every hue,
The pink, the violet, the white and the blue,
The chatty, the catty, the boring, the adoring,
The cold and official and the heart's outpouring,
Clever, stupid, short and long,
The typed and the printed and the spelt all wrong.

WH Auden

Matilda

Who Told Lies, and was Burned to Death

Matilda told such Dreadful Lies,
It made one Gasp and Stretch one's Eyes;
Her Aunt, who, from her Earliest Youth,
Had kept a Strict Regard for Truth,
Attempted to Believe Matilda:
The effort very nearly killed her,
And would have done so, had not She
Discovered this Infirmity.
For once, towards the Close of Day,
Matilda, growing tired of play,
And finding she was left alone,
Went tiptoe to the Telephone
And summoned the Immediate Aid
Of London's Noble Fire-Brigade.
Within an hour the Gallant Band
Were pouring in on every hand,
From Putney, Hackney Downs, and Bow
With Courage high and Hearts a-glow
They galloped, roaring through the Town
"Matilda's House is Burning Down!"
Inspired by British Cheers and Loud
Proceeding from the Frenzied Crowd,
They ran their ladders through a score
Of windows on the Ball Room Floor;
And took Peculiar Pains to Souse
The Pictures up and down the House,
Until Matilda's Aunt succeeded
In showing them they were not needed;
And even then she had to pay
To get the Men to go away!

Hilaire Belloc

PROSODY 1 D

The Owl and the Pussy-Cat

The Owl and the Pussy-Cat went to sea
   In a beautiful pea-green boat,
They took some honey, and plenty of money,
   Wrapped up in a five-pound note.
The Owl looked up to the stars above,
   And sang to a small guitar,
"O lovely Pussy! O Pussy, my love,
   What a beautiful Pussy you are,
      You are,
      You are!
   What a beautiful Pussy you are!"

Pussy said to the Owl, "You elegant fowl!
   How charmingly sweet you sing!
Oh let us be married! too long we have tarried:
   But what shall we do for a ring?"
They sailed away for a year and a day,
   To the land where the Bong-tree grows,
And there in a wood a Piggy-wig stood,
   With a ring at the end of his nose,
      His nose,
      His nose,
   With a ring at the end of his nose.

Edward Lear

The Old Sailor

There was an old sailor my grandfather knew
Who had so many things which he wanted to do
That, whenever he thought it was time to begin,
He couldn't because of the state he was in.

He was shipwrecked, and lived on an island for weeks,
And he wanted a hat, and he wanted some breeks;
And he wanted some nets, or a line and some hooks
For the turtles and things which you read of in books.

So he thought of his hut . . . and he thought of his boat,
And his hat and his breeks, and his chicken and goat,
And the hooks (for his food) and the spring (for his thirst) . . .
But he could never think which he ought to do first.

And so in the end he did nothing at all,
But basked on the shingle wrapped up in a shawl.
And I think it was dreadful the way he behaved —
He did nothing but basking until he was saved!

AA Milne

PROSODY 1 D

The Underground

      The Underground
      Goes round and round
And also to and fro;
      And men in blue
      Look after you
And tell you how to go.
      They never quite
      Direct you right,
Although, of course, they know.

      The Underground
      Goes round and round
And makes a lot of fuss;
      And men in blue
      Make fools of you,
Which is ridiculous.
      So that is why
      For my part I
Am sitting on a bus.

      The platform-man
      Has got a plan
For dealing with a queue;
      He makes men wait
      Behind a gate
Until their train is due;
      They watch their train
      Depart again,
And then he lets them through.

Guy Boas

A Subaltern's Love-Song

Miss J. Hunter Dunn, Miss J. Hunter Dunn,
Furnish'd and burnish'd by Aldershot sun,
What strenuous singles we played after tea,
We in the tournament — you against me!

Love-thirty, love-forty, oh! weakness of joy,
The speed of a swallow, the grace of a boy,
With carefullest carelessness, gaily you won,
I am weak from your loveliness, Joan Hunter Dunn.

Miss Joan Hunter Dunn, Miss Joan Hunter Dunn,
How mad I am, sad I am, glad that you won.
The warm-handled racket is back in its press,
But my shock-headed victor, she loves me no less.

The scent of the conifers, sound of the bath,
The view from my bedroom of moss-dappled path,
As I struggle with double-end evening tie,
For we dance at the Golf Club, my victor and I.

And the scent of her wrap, and the words never said,
And the ominous, ominous dancing ahead.
We sat in the car park till twenty to one
And now I'm engaged to Miss Joan Hunter Dunn.

John Betjeman

PROSODY I D

From a Railway Carriage

Faster than fairies, faster than witches,
Bridges and houses, hedges and ditches;
And charging along like troops in a battle,
All through the meadows the horses and cattle;
All of the sights of the hill and the plain
Fly as thick as driving rain;
And ever again, in the wink of an eye,
Painted stations whistle by.

Here is a child who clambers and scrambles,
All by himself and gathering brambles;
Here is a tramp who stands and gazes;
And there is the green for stringing daisies!
Here is a cart run away in the road
Lumping along with man and load;
And here is a mill, and there is a river:
Each a glimpse and gone for ever!

Robert Louis Stevenson

The Tiger

Tiger! Tiger! burning bright
In the forests of the night,
What immortal hand or eye
Could frame thy fearful symmetry?

In what distant deeps or skies
Burnt the fire of thine eyes?
On what wings dare he aspire?
What the hand dare seize the fire?

And what shoulder, and what art,
Could twist the sinews of thy heart?
And, when thy heart began to beat,
What dread hand? And what dread feet?

What the hammer? What the chain?
In what furnace was thy brain?
What the anvil? What dread grasp
Dare its deadly terrors clasp?

When the stars threw down their spears,
And watered heaven with their tears,
Did he smile his work to see?
Did he who made the Lamb make thee?

Tiger! Tiger! burning bright
In the forests of the night,
What immortal hand or eye
Dare frame thy fearful symmetry?

William Blake

PROSODY 1 D

The Charge of the Light Brigade

Half a league, half a league,
   Half a league onward,
All in the valley of Death
   Rode the six hundred.
"Forward, the Light Brigade!
Charge for the guns", he said:
Into the valley of Death
   Rode the six hundred.

"Forward, the Light Brigade!"
Was there a man dismayed?
Not though the soldier knew
   Some one had blundered:
Their's not to make reply,
Their's not to reason why,
Their's but to do and die:
Into the valley of Death
   Rode the six hundred.

Cannon to right of them,
Cannon to left of them,
Cannon in front of them
   Vollyed and thundered;
Stormed at with shot and shell,
Boldly they rode and well,
Into the jaws of Death,
Into the mouth of Hell
Rode the six hundred.

Alfred, Lord Tennyson

SECTION 5
PROSODY II

The exercises contained in this section have been designed to provide practice in a range of **intonation** drills. Examples of many different sentence types are given, together with a description of the normal intonation pattern. It is, of course, quite possible that therapists may wish to change the intonation pattern to convey different shades of meaning. The writers encourage therapists to do so, and recommend that a good clear model be given for the patient to imitate.

A	'Wh' questions	115
B	'Yes'/'No' questions	118
C	Simple declarative statements	120
D	'Tag' questions	122
E	'Change of mood' sentences to extend intonation range	123

'Wh' questions

A PROSODY II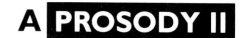

■ **High head, high fall nucleus**
  (falling intonation on stressed syllables)

▶ *'What' questions*

ˈWhat's the ˈtime?
ˈWhat's your ˈname?
ˈWhat will you ˈdo?
ˈWhat do you ˈwant?
ˈWhat will happen ˈnext?
ˈWhat did he ˈdo?
ˈWhat's that ˈtune?
ˈWhat time is the ˈkick-off?
ˈWhat's the name of the ˈfilm?
ˈWhat's his ˈtelephone number?

▶ *'Where' questions*

ˈWhere have you ˈbeen?
ˈWhere are you ˈgoing?
ˈWhere can it ˈbe?
ˈWhere will I ˈfind it?
ˈWhere have you left your ˈcase?
ˈWhere do you ˈlive?
ˈWhere did you park the ˈcar?
ˈWhere is the ˈtheatre?
ˈWhere is the ˈrailway station?
ˈWhere is Sam's ˈspanner?

PROSODY II A

▶ *'When' questions*

ˈWhen are you ˈleaving?
ˈWhen will he arrìve?
ˈWhen is your ˈbirthday?
ˈWhen can I ˈcall?
ˈWhen will it stop ˈraining?
ˈWhen did your ˈplane get in?
ˈWhen can you come aˈgain?
ˈWhen is ˈEaster this year?
ˈWhen does the ˈfilm begin?
ˈWhen will he leave the ˈhospital?

▶ *'Why' questions*

ˈWhy did it ˈhappen?
ˈWhy did you do ˈthat?
ˈWhy won't the ˈcar start?
ˈWhy must you ˈleave?
ˈWhy are you ˈsmiling?
ˈWhy is your ˈhair wet?
ˈWhy are you ˈlate?
ˈWhy don't you go ˈhome?
ˈWhy is she ˈcrying?
ˈWhy don't we ˈall go?

▶ *'Which' questions*

ˈWhich ˈdress will you wear?
ˈWhich is the ˈnearest shop?
ˈWhich answer is corˈrect?
ˈWhich way did he ˈgo?
ˈWhich one do you like ˈbest?
ˈWhich book do you recomˈmend?
ˈWhich ˈroad do I take?
ˈWhich bus goes into ˈtown?
ˈWhich bottle is ˈfull?
ˈWhich of the twins has ˈfair hair?

A PROSODY II

▶ *'Who' questions*

ˈWho gave you perˈmission?
ˈWho wrote this ˈpoem?
ˈWho's next in the ˈqueue?
ˈWho told ˈKen about it?
ˈWho said he wasn't ˈcoming?
ˈWho gave Jill the ˈanswer?
ˈWho drove the ˈcar home?
ˈWho's going to ˈLondon?
ˈWho arrived ˈyesterday?
ˈWho's staying at home with the ˈbaby?

▶ *'How' questions*

ˈHow are you ˈfeeling?
ˈHow did you ˈget here?
ˈHow many are ˈcoming?
ˈHow can you do ˈthat?
ˈHow is your ˈfriend?
ˈHow do you ˈknow?
ˈHow much is the ˈsweater?
ˈHow do you make ˈshortbread?
ˈHow long is he ˈstaying?
ˈHow clever is ˈJohn?

PROSODY II B   'Yes'/'No' questions

■ **High head, low rise nucleus (rising intonation on stressed syllable)**

▶ *'Yes'/'No' questions*

ˈAre you ˏangry?
ˈIs it ˏyour book?
ˈDo you take ˏsugar?
ˈDo you know him ˏwell?
ˈDo you like ˏtea?
ˈDo you ˏsmoke?
ˈDid you enjoy the ˏfilm?
ˈMay I have a ˏdrink?
ˈWill he be home ˏsoon?
ˈHave you any ˏcheese?

ˈMay I have some ˏbacon?
ˈAre these ˏyour things?
ˈWere you born in ˏFrance?
ˈWill you come to ˏtea?
ˈCan you ˏswim?
ˈHave you seen that ˏfilm?
ˈDid it ˏrain today?
ˈDo you have ˏa pet?
ˈHave you been to ˏschool?

ˈAre you ˏhungry?
ˈAre you ˏthirsty?
ˈAre you ˏangry?
ˈCan you ˏsee me?
ˈWill he be on ˏtime?
ˈIs the tap still ˏdripping?
ˈIs it too ˏlate?
ˈDid you see him ˏgo?
ˈDo you ˏlive here?
ˈWould you like a ˏsandwich?

ˈMay I ˌhelp you?
ˈIs Tom ˌyour son?
ˈDid your grandchildren come to ˌstay?
ˈAre you going aˌbroad for your holiday?
ˈDo you think he'll be eleˌcted?
ˈDo you like ˌwalking?
ˈDo you listen to the ˌradio?
ˈDo you read the ˌnewspaper?
ˈDo you watch teleˌvision?
ˈIs today ˌFriday?

ˈAre you going away for the ˌweek-end?
ˈHave you heard their latest ˌrecord?
ˈHave you ˌwritten to him yet?
ˈHave you sent John a ˌpostcard?
ˈAre you flying to ˌParis?

ˈIs Washington the capital of Aˌmerica?
ˈDid you have a good ˌjourney?
ˈDoes the performance start at ˌeight?
ˈHave you taken a ˌphotograph?
ˈIs your brother's name ˌBill?
ˈWill you come to ˌLondon with me?
ˈDid you enjoy the ˌmeal?

ˈWas it a good ˌstory?
ˈWill Bob be able to fix the ˌcar?
ˈWas there much traffic on the ˌmotorway?
ˈIs there fresh cream in this ˌcake?
ˈDid she telephone toˌday?
ˈDo you need your ˌovercoat?

PROSODY II C

Simple declarative statements

■ **Falling intonation starting on final stressed syllable**

My ˋfeet are hurting.
It's a ˋquarter to ten.
I'm ˋgoing to bed.
I ˋcame by bus.
I've ˋmade you a cake.
I ˋwant to go home.
Your ˋskirt is too long.
My ˋdress is old.
Her ˋfeet are hurting.
They came here by ˋtrain.

Its ˋtime for them to go.
It's ˋnever too late.
Her ˋcar is bright red.
Some people ˋnever learn.
The ˋengine won't start.
Today is ˋMonday.
Come with me in the ˋcar.
Let's make some ˋcakes.
Kate's car was in the ˋhigh street.
Your ˋdaughter gave me the book.

I've found the ˋmagazine you wanted.
Take the ˋdog out of here.
Mary's coat was very exˋpensive.
The referee's decision is ˋfinal.
We are looking for a flat for our reˋtirement.
Take your umˋbrella with you.
He's a stockbroker in the ˋcity.
Lemon tea is a ˋvery refreshing drink.
Yesterday we went for a ˋdrive.
Sign your name ˋhere, please.
Tangerines are in season ˋnow.
We pick strawberries in the ˋsummer.
It's a ˋnon-stick saucepan.
Let's call a taxi to take us to the ˋairport.

C PROSODY II

- **Falling intonation:** choose stressed syllable (and hence start of falling intonation according to the meaning you wish to convey.
  eg. ˋHe always reads the newspaper.
      He ˋalways reads the newspaper.
      He always reads the ˋnewspaper.

We can wash the dishes before the programme starts.
Look at the snow outside.
I'm sure he was in the shop earlier.
Children usually like ice-cream.
It's too dangerous to hitch-hike nowadays.
The rehearsal begins at seven-thirty.
He bought that record yesterday.

David has a meeting in London.
The train is due in half an hour.
The flight takes about two hours.
There will be a car waiting for you.
Bring a packed lunch with you.
Mint sauce is best with lamb.
The wind is blowing from the east.
The race ended in a dead-heat.
The dress was reduced to half-price.
I've bought four tickets for the show.

He's up in the balcony.
They're getting married next week.
Jill and Eric have bought a bungalow.
He is a confirmed bachelor.
There was a bad accident on the motorway.
The factory is closing next year.
John Smith would make a good president.
There is a general election next month.

PROSODY II D

'Tag' questions

- **Rising intonation on 'tag' implies doubt;**
- **Falling intonation on 'tag' implies certainty and that you are politely confirming the statement**

It's three o'clock, isn't it?
He went home, didn't he?
That's my car, isn't it?
You'll give it to him, won't you?
He'll drive you home, won't he?
He'd telephone you, wouldn't he?
You should go immediately, shouldn't you?
That's an amazing story, isn't it?
Sheila came to see you in hospital, didn't she?
He said he'd wash the car, didn't he?

They'll all be coming for dinner, won't they?
She should see a specialist, shouldn't she?
Ann will settle the argument, won't she?
The train leaves at five-thirty, doesn't it?
The central heating is too hot, isn't it?
They would go straight to Harry's, wouldn't they?
They should be saving their money, shouldn't they?
You can get in for nothing, can't you?
We can all smile for the camera, can't we?
He could go to the supermarket on the way home, couldn't he?
He goes to the office every day, doesn't he?
She rides a horse, doesn't she?

'Change of mood' sentences to extend intonation range

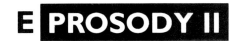

- By changing the stress and/or intonation it is possible to convey different meanings or moods.
- How many changes of mood or meaning can you convey in the following sentences?

I know about that.
What do you think?
Go on, tell me all about it.
You know I wanted to come.
I'm not sure about that.
When is all this going to end?
Don't tell anyone about it.
Twenty thousand people saw it happen.
He won a quarter of a million pounds.
When will she learn her lesson?

We could go tomorrow if you like.
What do you mean?
Why do you behave like this?
Whatever you say.
I really couldn't say.
Trust Ron to spill the beans.
Whose book is it anyway?
That's a very interesting point.
Has everyone heard the news?
I know what you say is true.

SECTION 6
PROSODY III

This section contains two short plays which can be acted out. They provide particular opportunities to practise stress and intonation.

The section also contains some ideas for role-play situations which will provide a bridge towards free spontaneous conversation.

Dialogue 1: **Keep to the Left!**

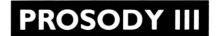

- **A policeman**
- **A visitor to England**

▶ *A street in an English town. A policeman stops a car. In the car there is a visitor from another country.*

POLICEMAN: (*holding up his hand*) Stop!
VISITOR: (*in car*) What's the matter?
POLICEMAN: Why are you driving on the right side of the road?
VISITOR: Do you want me to drive on the wrong side?
POLICEMAN: You are driving on the wrong side.
VISITOR: But you said that I was driving on the right side.
POLICEMAN: That's right. You're on the right, and that's wrong.
VISITOR: A strange country! If right is wrong, I'm right when I'm on the wrong side. So why did you stop me?
POLICEMAN: My dear sir, you must keep to the left. The right side is the left.
VISITOR: It's like a looking-glass! I'll try to remember. Well, I want to go to Bellwood. Will you kindly tell me the way?
POLICEMAN: Certainly. At the end of this road, turn left.
VISITOR: Now let me think. Turn left! In England left is right and right is wrong. Am I right?
POLICEMAN: You'll be right if you turn left. But if you turn right, you'll be wrong.
VISITOR: Thank you. It's as clear as daylight.

PROSODY III

Dialogue 2: **No Time to Waste**

- **Doctor Vine, a busy doctor**
- **Mr Lester, one of his friends**

▶ *Doctor Vine is busy at a desk with some papers. Lester runs into the room. He has black marks on his face and hands.*

VINE: This is the wrong time of the day to come and see me.

LESTER: I just wanted to —

VINE: Everyone always 'just wants' something or other. I'm going out. What have you done to your face and hands? Have you had a fight with someone? At your age? You mustn't do that kind of thing. How's your heart? I'll just listen to it. Take your coat off.

LESTER: But you don't need to do that.

VINE: Oh, yes, I do. Are you trying to teach me my business? Take your coat off at once.

LESTER: I won't.

VINE: Oh, yes, you will. Take your coat off when I tell you. I know my own business best, and I've no time to waste.

LESTER: I won't take it off. I only want —

VINE: If you don't take it off, I will. I'm a busy man. (*He pulls LESTER'S coat off.*) Now sit down there on that chair.

LESTER: You don't understand. I just want —

VINE: Sit down and don't talk. (*He pulls LESTER down on the chair.*) That's better. Now don't move.

LESTER: But —

VINE: And don't talk. How can I listen to your heart when you're talking? (*Listens*) Hm! Hm! I don't like this at all. Does your heart always go as fast as this? You must take a long rest, my dear Lester. No more work for you and no more parties for six months.

LESTER: (*putting his coat on*) I'm sorry to hear that. I came here to ask you to come to a party at my house next week. And when I reached your house, I found that it was on fire. I just wanted to tell you.

C PROSODY II

- **Falling intonation:** choose stressed syllable (and hence start of falling intonation according to the meaning you wish to convey.
  eg. ˋHe always reads the newspaper.
  He ˋalways reads the newspaper.
  He always reads the ˋnewspaper.

We can wash the dishes before the programme starts.
Look at the snow outside.
I'm sure he was in the shop earlier.
Children usually like ice-cream.
It's too dangerous to hitch-hike nowadays.
The rehearsal begins at seven-thirty.
He bought that record yesterday.

David has a meeting in London.
The train is due in half an hour.
The flight takes about two hours.
There will be a car waiting for you.
Bring a packed lunch with you.
Mint sauce is best with lamb.
The wind is blowing from the east.
The race ended in a dead-heat.
The dress was reduced to half-price.
I've bought four tickets for the show.

He's up in the balcony.
They're getting married next week.
Jill and Eric have bought a bungalow.
He is a confirmed bachelor.
There was a bad accident on the motorway.
The factory is closing next year.
John Smith would make a good president.
There is a general election next month.

PROSODY II D

'Tag' questions

- **Rising intonation on 'tag' implies doubt;**
- **Falling intonation on 'tag' implies certainty and that you are politely confirming the statement**

It's three o'clock, isn't it?
He went home, didn't he?
That's my car, isn't it?
You'll give it to him, won't you?
He'll drive you home, won't he?
He'd telephone you, wouldn't he?
You should go immediately, shouldn't you?
That's an amazing story, isn't it?
Sheila came to see you in hospital, didn't she?
He said he'd wash the car, didn't he?

They'll all be coming for dinner, won't they?
She should see a specialist, shouldn't she?
Ann will settle the argument, won't she?
The train leaves at five-thirty, doesn't it?
The central heating is too hot, isn't it?
They would go straight to Harry's, wouldn't they?
They should be saving their money, shouldn't they?
You can get in for nothing, can't you?
We can all smile for the camera, can't we?
He could go to the supermarket on the way home, couldn't he?
He goes to the office every day, doesn't he?
She rides a horse, doesn't she?

'Change of mood' sentences to extend intonation range

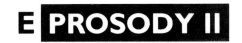

- By changing the stress and/or intonation it is possible to convey different meanings or moods.
- How many changes of mood or meaning can you convey in the following sentences?

I know about that.
What do you think?
Go on, tell me all about it.
You know I wanted to come.
I'm not sure about that.
When is all this going to end?
Don't tell anyone about it.
Twenty thousand people saw it happen.
He won a quarter of a million pounds.
When will she learn her lesson?

We could go tomorrow if you like.
What do you mean?
Why do you behave like this?
Whatever you say.
I really couldn't say.
Trust Ron to spill the beans.
Whose book is it anyway?
That's a very interesting point.
Has everyone heard the news?
I know what you say is true.

SECTION 6
PROSODY III

This section contains two short plays which can be acted out. They provide particular opportunities to practise stress and intonation.

The section also contains some ideas for role-play situations which will provide a bridge towards free spontaneous conversation.

Dialogue I: **Keep to the Left!**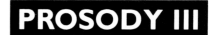

- **A policeman**
- **A visitor to England**

▶ *A street in an English town. A policeman stops a car. In the car there is a visitor from another country.*

POLICEMAN: (*holding up his hand*) Stop!

VISITOR: (*in car*) What's the matter?

POLICEMAN: Why are you driving on the right side of the road?

VISITOR: Do you want me to drive on the wrong side?

POLICEMAN: You are driving on the wrong side.

VISITOR: But you said that I was driving on the right side.

POLICEMAN: That's right. You're on the right, and that's wrong.

VISITOR: A strange country! If right is wrong, I'm right when I'm on the wrong side. So why did you stop me?

POLICEMAN: My dear sir, you must keep to the left. The right side is the left.

VISITOR: It's like a looking-glass! I'll try to remember. Well, I want to go to Bellwood. Will you kindly tell me the way?

POLICEMAN: Certainly. At the end of this road, turn left.

VISITOR: Now let me think. Turn left! In England left is right and right is wrong. Am I right?

POLICEMAN: You'll be right if you turn left. But if you turn right, you'll be wrong.

VISITOR: Thank you. It's as clear as daylight.

PROSODY III

Dialogue 2: **No Time to Waste**

- **Doctor Vine, a busy doctor**
- **Mr Lester, one of his friends**

▶ *Doctor Vine is busy at a desk with some papers. Lester runs into the room. He has black marks on his face and hands.*

VINE: This is the wrong time of the day to come and see me.

LESTER: I just wanted to —

VINE: Everyone always 'just wants' something or other. I'm going out. What have you done to your face and hands? Have you had a fight with someone? At your age? You mustn't do that kind of thing. How's your heart? I'll just listen to it. Take your coat off.

LESTER: But you don't need to do that.

VINE: Oh, yes, I do. Are you trying to teach me my business? Take your coat off at once.

LESTER: I won't.

VINE: Oh, yes, you will. Take your coat off when I tell you. I know my own business best, and I've no time to waste.

LESTER: I won't take it off. I only want —

VINE: If you don't take it off, I will. I'm a busy man. (*He pulls LESTER'S coat off.*) Now sit down there on that chair.

LESTER: You don't understand. I just want —

VINE: Sit down and don't talk. (*He pulls LESTER down on the chair.*) That's better. Now don't move.

LESTER: But —

VINE: And don't talk. How can I listen to your heart when you're talking? (*Listens*) Hm! Hm! I don't like this at all. Does your heart always go as fast as this? You must take a long rest, my dear Lester. No more work for you and no more parties for six months.

LESTER: (*putting his coat on*) I'm sorry to hear that. I came here to ask you to come to a party at my house next week. And when I reached your house, I found that it was on fire. I just wanted to tell you.

Role-play

PROSODY III

■ It is suggested that therapist and patient(s) change roles when acting out these situations.

TV interview: Pretend you are appearing on a TV 'chat' show and being interviewed.

Pretend you are giving an account of an accident or fire you have witnessed, to a **local newspaper reporter**, for example.

Restaurant scene: Imagine you are ordering a snack or meal in a restaurant.

Restaurant scene: Pretend that you are unhappy with the meal you have been served and make complaints.

Shopping: Imagine that you wish to make an expensive purchase, such as an item of furniture, TV, stereo, washing machine, computer or camera. You should ask a number of detailed, searching questions of the sales assistant.

Shopping: You have bought an article, in recent weeks/months which has proved to be unsatisfactory. Act out the scene when you return the article and complain.

Buying railway, airline, theatre tickets: Pretend you are at the booking office making your purchase or on the telephone trying to make the bookings.

Travel agency scene: Imagine you are in a travel agency and you wish to book a holiday.

Estate agent: Pretend that you have come into an estate agent's office and wish to buy a house. You may be new to the district; you may ask to be taken to see a property and so on.

Car salesman: Pretend that you wish to buy either a new or a second-hand car. Be ready to ask lots of awkward questions if you are the customer, or be ready with good answers if you are the salesman.

Garage scene: Pretend that your car has a mechanical problem and you wish to have it repaired, serviced and so on.

Discussion time: Discuss topical issues such as the cost of living, local building plans, motorway traffic, discipline in schools, public transport and so on.

ALPHABET CHART

A	B	C	D	E	F	G	H
I	J	K	L	M	N	O	P
Q	R	S	T	U	V	W	X
Y	Z	.	1	2	3	4	5
6	7	8	9	0	£	$	?

a	b	c	d	e	f	g	h
i	j	k	l	m	n	o	p
q	r	s	t	u	v	w	x
y	z	.	1	2	3	4	5
6	7	8	9	0	£	$	?

ACKNOWLEDGEMENTS

The authors and publishers wish to thank the following for permission to reproduce copyright material:

p99	Nash Publishing Corporation (USA) for lines from 'Do You Have It In A 60 Extra-Long?' from *It Could Be Verse* by Victor Buono (1972).
pps99–100	Faber & Faber Ltd for the complete 'The Rum Tum Tugger' from TS Eliot's *Old Possum's Book of Practical Cats* (1972).
p101	Nash Publishing Corporation (USA) for lines from 'A Fat Man's Prayer' from *It Could Be Verse* by Victor Buono (1972).
p103	The Society of Authors as the literary representative of the Estate of John Masefield for extracts from 'Cargoes' and 'Sea-Fever' from *Poems* by John Masefield.
p104	Faber & Faber Ltd for extracts from 'Night Mail' from *Collected Poems* by WH Auden.
p105	Peters Fraser & Dunlop Group Ltd for extracts from 'Matilda' from *Cautionary Verses* by Hilaire Belloc.
p109	John Murray (Publishers) Ltd for extracts from 'A Subaltern's Love-Song' from *The Collected Poems*, John Betjeman (1979).